Registered Dietitian Exam
Practice Questions

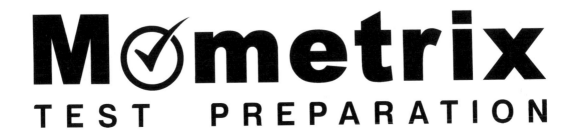

DEAR FUTURE EXAM SUCCESS STORY

First of all, **THANK YOU** for purchasing Mometrix study materials!

Second, congratulations! You are one of the few determined test-takers who are committed to doing whatever it takes to excel on your exam. **You have come to the right place.** We developed these practice tests with one goal in mind: to deliver you the best possible approximation of the questions you will see on test day.

Standardized testing is one of the biggest obstacles on your road to success, which only increases the importance of doing well in the high-pressure, high-stakes environment of test day. Your results on this test could have a significant impact on your future, and these practice tests will give you the repetitions you need to build your familiarity and confidence with the test content and format to help you achieve your full potential on test day.

Your success is our success

We would love to hear from you! If you would like to share the story of your exam success or if you have any questions or comments in regard to our products, please contact us at **800-673-8175** or **support@mometrix.com**.

Thanks again for your business and we wish you continued success!

Sincerely,
The Mometrix Test Preparation Team

TABLE OF CONTENTS

Practice Test #1

1. Which of the following carbohydrates is not a monosaccharide?

a. Fructose
b. Galactose
c. Maltose
d. Glucose

2. Which of the following statements about glycogen is TRUE?

a. Glycogen is a long-term energy source.
b. The liver stores approximately 100 grams of glycogen.
c. Glycogen is stored primarily in the liver but also appears in skeletal and heart muscles.
d. The glycogen found in skeletal muscles is catabolized for use anywhere in the body.

3. Which of the following statements about controlling blood glucose levels is FALSE?

a. Beta cells in the islets of Langerhans produce insulin, which is released when blood glucose levels rise in response to a meal.
b. Alpha cells in the islets of Langerhans secrete glucagon when the patient is fasting, which stimulates the liver to break down glycogen to maintain blood glucose levels in the normal range of 80-100 mg/dL.
c. The adrenal glands secrete epinephrine and norepinephrine when a patient is fasting, which stimulates muscles to release glycogen to maintain blood glucose levels.
d. Glucocorticoids, such as cortisol, stimulate glycolysis to increase blood glucose levels.

4. Body fat performs all of the following functions EXCEPT:

a. Providing a concentrated source of energy
b. Protecting bones and internal organs by cushioning them and regulating their temperature
c. Providing a source of eicosapentaenoic (EPA) and docosahexaenoic (DHA) essential fatty acids
d. Aiding in the absorption of the fat-soluble vitamins A, D, E, and K

5. Which of the following are not essential amino acids?

a. Lysine, leucine, valine
b. Isoleucine, tryptophan, phenylalanine
c. Methionine, threonine, lysine
d. Tyrosine, glycine, alanine

6. Which of the following statements about excessive protein intake is FALSE?

a. Excessive protein intake is difficult to achieve and, therefore, is not a danger.
b. Excessive protein intake increases calcium excretion, which can potentially lead to osteoporosis.
c. Excessive protein in the diet is broken down in the kidneys and excreted in the urine as urea.
d. Excessive protein intake will not help an athlete build more muscles, but will instead convert into fat, if it is not used as an energy source.

1

7. How many grams of protein are in a meal containing 6 ounces baked fish, 1 cup cooked pasta, 1 cup steamed broccoli, 1 slice whole wheat bread, 1 cup skim milk, 1/2 cup sliced strawberries, and 1 slice angel cake?

    a. 54 grams
    b. 66 grams
    c. 75 grams
    d. 83 grams

8. Kwashiorkor patients have all of the following characteristics EXCEPT:

    a. loss of somatic stores.
    b. a lack of amino acids.
    c. loss of visceral protein stores.
    d. a large, protruding abdomen.

9. Which description of marasmus is the most accurate?

    a. Starvation from food deprivation, with a decrease in somatic and visceral proteins stores, but subcutaneous fat stores are preserved.
    b. Protein deprivation, with adequate calories from carbohydrates and depletion of visceral protein stores, but preservation of somatic stores.
    c. Severe malnutrition, with loss of subcutaneous fat and depletion of muscle mass, followed by a breakdown in lean body mass.
    d. A form of malnutrition mainly seen in the United States, due to limited access to food.

10. Which of the following statements about Vitamin D is FALSE?

    a. Vitamin D is activated by two hydroxylations; the first hydroxylation occurs in the liver and the second hydroxylation occurs in the kidneys.
    b. The most active form of Vitamin D occurs after hydroxylation in the kidney to 1, 25-dihydroxyvitamin D, also known as calcitriol.
    c. The most active form of Vitamin D is 25-hydroxycholecalciferol and occurs after hydroxylation in the liver.
    d. The main function of Vitamin D is calcium and phosphorus homeostasis.

11. All of the following foods are good sources of niacin EXCEPT:

    a. chicken.
    b. tuna.
    c. mushrooms.
    d. baked potato.

12. Which of the following statements about zinc absorption is TRUE?

    a. Zinc absorption is lower during pregnancy and lactation.
    b. Consuming a high-protein meal promotes zinc absorption through the formation of zinc-amino acid chelates, a more easily absorbed form of zinc
    c. Both phytates and tannins affect zinc absorption.
    d. Consuming soy protein inhibits zinc absorption.

13. Which of the following statements best describes a normal infant's growth during the first year of life?

 a. An infant loses weight initially after birth, regains it by day 10, doubles birth weight by 6 months, and triples birth weight and doubles length by his/her first birthday.

 b. An infant loses weight initially after birth, regains it by day 10, doubles birth weight by 4 months, and quadruples weight and triples length during the first year.

 c. After birth, the growth of an infant depends solely on the nutrition he/she receives.

 d. The growth percentiles determined at birth are the best predictor of the infant's growth during infancy and childhood.

14. Physiologic changes in an older person may include all of the following EXCEPT:

 a. a loss of lean body mass and an increase in adipose tissue.

 b. a loss of kidney function from age 30, due to gradual loss of nephrons and reduced blood flow.

 c. up to 40% reduction in resting metabolic rate, due to reduced lean body mass, since muscle is the most metabolically active tissue.

 d. achlorhydria, resulting in a Vitamin B_{12} deficiency, because stomach acid is required to absorb Vitamin B_{12}.

15. A very young child is at highest risk for a deficiency in:

 a. protein.

 b. vitamin C.

 c. calcium.

 d. iron.

16. Which of the following statements most accurately describes nutrition screening?

 a. A registered dietitian must complete nutrition screening.

 b. The purpose of a nutrition screen is to identify people with malnutrition or who are high-risk for developing malnutrition.

 c. The elderly population benefits most from nutrition screening.

 d. A proper nutritional screen requires the patient's height, weight, and laboratory data.

17. The Nutrition Screening Initiative is a joint project between all of the following groups EXCEPT the:

 a. American Dietetic Association.

 b. American Academy of Family Physicians.

 c. National Council on Aging.

 d. American Medical Association.

18. The Nutrition Screening Initiative uses a checklist with the acronym DETERMINE, which stands for:

a. **D**ental problems, **E**ating Poorly, **T**ransportation issues, **E**conomic Hardship, **R**educed Social Contact, **M**ultiple Medicines, **I**nvoluntary Weight Loss/Gain, **N**eeds Assistance in Self-Care, **E**lder Years Above Age 80.

b. **D**isease, **E**ating Problems, **T**ransportation Issues, **E**conomic Hardship, **R**educed Mobility, **M**ultiple Medicines, **I**nvoluntary Weight Loss/Gain, **N**eeds Assistance in Self-Care, **E**lder Years Above Age 80.

c. **D**isease, **E**ating Poorly, **T**ooth Loss/Mouth Pain, **E**conomic Hardship, **R**educed Social Contact, **M**ultiple Medicines, **I**nvoluntary Weight Loss/Gain, **N**eeds Assistance in Self-Care, **E**lder Years Above Age 80.

d. **D**isease, **E**ating Problems, **T**ooth Loss/Mouth Pain, **E**xtreme Difficulty with Mobility, **R**educed Gastrointestinal Function, **M**ultiple Medicines, **I**nvoluntary Weight Loss/Gain, **N**eeds Assistance in Self-Care, **E**lder Years Above Age 80.

19. Which of the following programs do not incorporate a nutrition screening as part of the enrollment process?

a. The Head Start Program
b. Special Supplemental Nutrition Program for Women, Infants, and Children (WIC)
c. Farmer's Market Nutrition Program
d. Supplemental Nutrition Assistance Program

20. The Mini Nutritional Assessment (MNA) is:

a. a validated nutrition screening and assessment tool to identify the presence or risk of malnutrition in patients 65 and older.
b. a validated nutrition screening and assessment tool to identify malnutrition in infants and children.
c. a nutrition screening tool used to enroll elderly patients into appropriate food assistance programs.
d. a nutrition screening tool that identifies children and their families who require enrollment into food assistance programs.

21. The National Health and Nutrition Examination Survey (NHANES) is:

a. a federal screening program that interviews 10,000 Americans each year to determine their medical and dental histories.
b. a state program that examines people over the age of 18 to gather their health-related information (demographic, socioeconomic, and nutritional).
c. a state program that obtains information from participants to improve health promotion and epidemiological research.
d. a federal program that combines an interview with a physical exam to assess the general health and nutritional status of participants of any age living in the United States.

22. All of the following statements about Healthy People 2030 are true EXCEPT:

a. the key goals are to increase the quality of life and the number of years spent in good health, and to eliminate disparities in health.
b. there are 355 objectives set to meet by 2030.
c. the program originated in the 1960s through the Surgeon General's Report on Health Promotion and Disease Prevention
d. there are 62 topic areas divide across five categories.

23. Data obtained for the Nutrition Assessment piece of the Nutrition Care Process is organized into which of the following five categories?

a. Food/nutrition-related history; laboratory data and medical tests; social history; nutrition-focused physical findings; and client history

b. Food/nutrition-related history; laboratory data; anthropometric measurements; physician exam; and client history

c. Food/nutrition-related history; biochemical data and medical tests; anthropometric measurements; nutrition-focused physical findings; and client history

d. Diet history; biochemical data and medical tests; anthropometric measurements; nutrition-focused physical findings; and medical exam findings

24. Which of the following categories is not represented in the Nutrition Diagnosis portion of the Nutrition Care Process?

a. Nutrition-focused etiology
b. Intake
c. Clinical
d. Behavioral/Environmental

25. Critical thinking skills the dietitian requires to evaluate the PES statement in the Nutrition Care Process require:

a. evaluating which nutrition diagnosis to use for a patient and selecting the broadest scope to maximize impact.

b. evaluating the etiology, determining if the best "root cause" has been identified, and determining if the signs and symptoms can at least be improved with nutrition intervention.

c. evaluating changes in the patient's signs and symptoms, but using clinical judgment to ultimately determine the appropriate resolution for the nutritional diagnosis.

d. selecting the nutrition diagnosis most likely to be treated quickly and efficiently, with a clear resolution of symptoms.

26. Which of the following statements concerning medical and nutrition diagnoses is TRUE?

a. The physician determines the medical diagnosis, while the RD determines the nutrition diagnosis.
b. The physician must determine both the medical diagnosis and the nutrition diagnosis.
c. The medical diagnosis and the nutrition diagnosis must be identical.
d. The nutrition diagnosis cannot be resolved unless the medical diagnosis is also resolved.

27. A patient is a 65-year-old man, diagnosed with heart disease. He lives alone and has limited cooking skills. He frequents fast food restaurants because they are within walking distance of his house. He is 20 pounds overweight, with a BMI of 26. Which of the following is an appropriate PES based on the information gathered?

a. Heart disease related to fast food consumption, as evidenced by diet history
b. Excessive energy intake related to limited cooking skills, as evidenced by obesity
c. Excessive energy intake related to frequent consumption of fast food, as evidenced by BMI and diet history
d. Inadequate exercise related to heart disease, as evidenced by BMI and weight gain

28. A referral patient is a 52-year-old female with elevated glucose levels, diagnosed with diabetes mellitus. Her fasting blood glucose level is 132 mg/dL. Her BMI is 28, which has increased from 25 over the past several months. She performs physical exercise two or three times per week for approximately 15 minutes. Which of the following are the most accurate possible nutrition diagnoses?

   a. Excessive carbohydrate intake, physical inactivity, or diabetes mellitus
   b. Inappropriate carbohydrate intake, inadequate physical activity, or excessive energy intake
   c. Excessive carbohydrate intake, impaired nutrient utilization, or diabetes mellitus
   d. Altered nutrition-related lab values, physical inactivity, or overweight/obesity

29. A patient is a 46-year-old man, who is 6 feet tall and weighs 160 pounds. He presents with difficulty swallowing and weight loss of 20 pounds. He states he usually weighs 180 pounds. He has a long history of cigarette smoking but no other medical issues. The doctor admits the patient to the hospital to evaluate him for possible esophageal cancer. Admission blood work reveals a serum albumin of 2.8 g/dL. During the nutrition interview, his diet history shows that he consumes approximately 1,500 calories per day and has altered his diet to soft/semi-soft consistency to accommodate his dysphagia. Based on the above information, all of the following are possible nutrition diagnoses EXCEPT:

   a. inadequate energy intake.
   b. excessive smoking.
   c. swallowing difficulty (dysphagia).
   d. involuntary weight loss.

30. Which of the following dietary methodologies may the registered dietitian use when conducting a dietary history?

   a. Retrospective data collection, such as food frequency or 24-hour recall
   b. Prospective data collection, such as food frequency or food record
   c. Retrospective data collection, such calorie count or 24-hour recall
   d. Both retrospective data collection, such as food frequency or 24-hour recall, and prospective data collection, such as food record or food diary

31. Positive nitrogen balance occurs in:

   a. pregnant women.
   b. normal, healthy adults.
   c. an elderly person who is confined to bed.
   d. starvation.

32. Which of the following is a positive acute-phase protein?

   a. Albumin
   b. C-reactive protein
   c. Retinol-binding protein
   d. Transferrin

33. All of the following statements about serum albumin are true EXCEPT:
   a. the half-life of albumin is approximately 20 days.
   b. albumin is a negative acute-phase reactant that responds slowly to changes in nutritional status.
   c. measuring serum albumin is a valuable tool in assessing short-term changes in protein status.
   d. serum albumin levels decrease during infection.

34. Which of the following statements about homocysteine levels and cardiovascular disease (CVD) is FALSE?
   a. High homocysteine is an independent risk factor for developing CVD.
   b. A patient with low homocysteine has an increased risk of developing CVD.
   c. Supplementation with folate, Vitamin B_6 and Vitamin B_{12} will improve homocysteine levels, thus reducing the risk of CVD.
   d. Homocysteine levels are affected by diet.

35. Metabolic syndrome can be identified by the presence of:
   a. central obesity (waist circumference greater than 40 inches for men, 35 for women), fasting glucose levels greater than or equal to 100 mg/dL, and blood pressure greater than 130/85 mmHg.
   b. central obesity (waist circumference greater than 40 inches for men, 35 for women), blood pressure greater than 130/90 mmHg, and fasting glucose greater than 110 mg/dL.
   c. central obesity (waist circumference greater than 40 inches for men, 35 for women), serum triglyceride levels greater than or equal to 150 mg/dL, and HDL cholesterol level less than 35 mg/dL for men and 45 or less for women.
   d. serum triglyceride levels greater than or equal to 150 mg/dL, blood pressure greater than 130/85 mmHg, and fasting glucose levels greater than or equal to 120 mg/dL

36. Which of the following best describes the nutritional care for dumping syndrome?
   a. Small frequent meals with high protein, moderately fatty foods; limited concentrated sweets; and drinking liquids separately from meals
   b. Three moderately sized meals and three snacks containing moderate protein and fat, lactose-free foods, and fluids limited to 4 ounces per meal
   c. Small, frequent meals with high protein, low fat, and high fiber foods; ingesting liquids and concentrated sweets separately from meals; avoiding foods containing lactose
   d. Three moderately sized meals and three snacks with moderate protein, low fat, and low fiber; liquids limited to 4 ounces per meal; concentrated sweets limited to one or two servings per day

37. Crohn's disease and ulcerative colitis are the two main forms of inflammatory bowel disease (IBD). All of the following are true about IBD EXCEPT:
   a. the average age of onset for IBD is 15-30 years old, and IBD occurs equally in both males and females.
   b. nutrition is a major issue for both Crohn's disease and ulcerative colitis patients; however, malnutrition is likely to be more of a lifelong concern for patients with ulcerative colitis.
   c. Crohn's disease can present in any part of the GI tract; however, it most frequently involves the distal ileum and the colon.
   d. ulcerative colitis involves the colon and is a continuous disease.

38. Which of the following must the dietitian consider to assess the nutritional status of a patient with end-stage liver disease accurately?
   a. Nitrogen balance studies
   b. Creatinine height index
   c. Anthropometric data including information on weight changes and visual assessment
   d. Serum albumin level

39. Which statement best describes protein requirements in liver disease?
   a. In uncomplicated hepatitis or cirrhosis without encephalopathy, protein requirements are 1.0-1.2 grams per kilogram of actual weight to promote nitrogen balance.
   b. In uncomplicated hepatitis or cirrhosis without encephalopathy, protein requirements are 1.0-1.2 grams per kilogram of dry weight to promote nitrogen balance.
   c. A protein restriction of less than 0.6 grams per kilogram is recommended for acute encephalopathy.
   d. Protein requirements for most patients with compensated liver disease are 1.5-2.0 grams per kilogram.

40. The initial treatment for acute pancreatitis is to allow the pancreas to rest and:
   a. provide IV fluids for hydration until the patient is pain-free and nausea and vomiting have resolved. Initiate a clear liquid diet and gradually advance to a soft, low-fat diet based on patient tolerance.
   b. initiate parenteral nutrition immediately. When the patient is pain-free and nausea and vomiting have resolved, initiate a clear liquid diet. Gradually advance to a soft, low-fat diet based on patient tolerance.
   c. initiate enteral feeding immediately, using a defined formula fed into the jejunum. When the patient is stable, initiate a clear liquid diet. Slowly advance to a soft, low-fat diet.
   d. initiate a clear liquid diet when the patient's pain has subsided. Advance to a soft, low-fat diet with supplemental pancreatic enzymes to improve tolerance.

41. Which best describes the main priorities of medical nutrition therapy for Type I diabetes?
   a. Weight loss and meal planning
   b. Meal planning that incorporates the individual's usual eating and exercise habits, followed by development of an insulin regimen
   c. Implementation of a three-meal per day and two snack-meal plan, tailored to the insulin regimen already established
   d. Adjustment of usual eating habits to reflect an even carbohydrate distribution and initiation of regular exercise pattern, followed by development of an insulin regimen

42. All of the following goals are appropriate medical nutrition therapy for diabetes EXCEPT:
   a. maintain blood glucose levels as close to the normal range as possible to help prevent or delay complications of diabetes.
   b. adjust nutrient intake to help address possible complications resulting from obesity, heart disease, and nephropathy.
   c. learn to make healthier food choices and improve physical activity level to help improve overall health status.
   d. modify fat intake to help prevent the development of cardiovascular disease and improve lipid panel; modify protein intake to help prevent the development of nephropathy and other kidney-related complications.

43. Which of the following statements is the best advice the registered dietitian can give a diabetic patient regarding alcohol intake?

    a. Both men and women should limit their alcohol intake to one drink per day.

    b. Limit your alcohol consumption to 2 oz on an empty stomach, as alcohol increases blood glucose levels.

    c. Alcohol is an energy source that is not converted to glucose, unlike food. Alcohol inhibits gluconeogenesis, which can lead to hypoglycemia if you drink alcohol on an empty stomach.

    d. Alcohol is metabolized quickly; therefore, your risk of low blood glucose is lower if you consume alcohol after exercise.

44. Which of the following statements about intermediate acting insulin is TRUE?

    a. The onset of action is 30-60 minutes, peak action is 6-10 hours, and the duration is 10-16 hours.

    b. The onset of action is 15-30 minutes, peak action is 2-3 hours, and the duration is 6-8 hours.

    c. The onset of action is 4-6 hours, peak action is 10-12 hours, and the duration is 16-20 hours.

    d. The onset of action is 2-4 hours, peak action is 6-10 hours, and the duration is 10-16 hours.

45. When discussing sick day guidelines with a diabetic patient, the registered dietitian would include all of the following instructions EXCEPT:

    a. continue to take insulin as ordered by your physician, because your insulin requirements may increase due to sickness causing fever or stress.

    b. consume only sugar-free fluids to prevent hyperglycemia from an excessive sugar intake.

    c. consume adequate fluids, especially if you vomit. Drink 1 ounce every 15-30 minutes in small sips.

    d. check your blood glucose levels and your urine ketones at least 4 times daily. Call your doctor if ketones appear or if your blood glucose level is greater than 240 mg/dL.

46. Which of the following is the appropriate treatment for hypoglycemia?

    a. If the patient's blood glucose level is less than 70 mg/dL, give 4 ounces of juice or 1 tablespoon of sugar. Recheck the patient's blood glucose level in 15 minutes. If the level remains less than 70 mg/dL, give another 15 grams of carbohydrate.

    b. If the patient's blood glucose level is less than 70 mg/dL, give 8 ounces of juice or 6 glucose tablets. Recheck the blood glucose level in 30 minutes. If the level remains less than 70 mg/dL, give another 15-30 grams of carbohydrate.

    c. If the patient's blood glucose level is less than 70 mg/dL, give 8 ounces of juice or 4 glucose tablets. Recheck the blood glucose level in 30 minutes. If the level remains less than 70 mg/dL, give another 15-30 grams of carbohydrate.

    d. If the patient's blood glucose level is less than 70 mg/dL, give 8 ounces of juice or 10-12 Lifesavers. Recheck the blood glucose level in 15 minutes. If the level remains less than 70 mg/dL, give another 15-30 grams of carbohydrate.

47. Which of the following is the best description of cardiac risk, according to the ATP III guidelines of the National Cholesterol Education Program (NCEP)?

a. The HDL level is the primary marker, followed by the presence of any type of atherosclerotic disease, such as coronary heart disease, carotid artery disease, or peripheral arterial disease, and risk factors (smoking, hypertension, LDL levels greater than 100 mg/dL, age greater than 45, or significant family history).

b. The LDL cholesterol level is the primary marker, followed by the presence of coronary heart disease, and risk factors (smoking, hypertension, HDL levels less than 40 mg/dL, age greater than 45, or significant family history).

c. The total cholesterol level is the primary marker, followed by the presence of coronary heart disease, and risk factors, such as smoking, hypertension, HDL levels less than 40 mg/dL, age greater than 45, or significant family history.

d. The patient's total number of risk factors are significant for ATP III, such as: Smoking; hypertension; LDL level less than 40 mg/dL; total cholesterol greater than 240 mg/dL; family history, especially heart disease in a first-degree male family member younger than age 55; diabetes; and age (men older than 45 and women older than 55).

48. The American Heart Association's healthy eating recommendations for children to prevent heart disease indicates that a child must have:

a. a nutritious diet containing a variety of food groups; less than 35% of total calories from fat intake and less than 10% from saturated fat; cholesterol intake less than 300 mg per day; sufficient calorie intake to promote normal growth and development, but if the child is overweight, adjust calories to promote slow weight loss.

b. a nutritious diet containing a variety of food groups; total fat intake less than 30% of total calories; caloric intake tailored to achieve a healthy body weight, while maintaining normal growth and development; limited juice intake; and low fat or fat-free dairy products.

c. a nutritious diet containing a variety of food groups; total fat intake of 25-35% of total calories for children older than 4; mostly monounsaturated or polyunsaturated fat; five fruits and vegetables per day; whole grain products whenever possible; low fat or fat-free dairy products for children older than 2; and at least one hour of exercise most days of the week.

d. a nutritious diet containing a variety of food groups; total fat intake of 25-35% of total calories for children older than 2; sufficient calorie intake to promote normal growth and development; and 30 minutes per day of exercise. Monitor the overweight child, who will likely grow into the weight as height increases.

49. The dietitian who begins nutrition therapy for a cardiovascular disease patient realizes the outcome measures are influenced most by:

a. family history, age, gender, socioeconomic status, and cigarette smoking.

b. HDL cholesterol, dietary modifications, and LDL cholesterol.

c. oxidative stress, triglycerides, HDL cholesterol, and total cholesterol.

d. obesity, physical activity, and thrombogenic factors, such as fibrinogen.

50. The Therapeutic Lifestyle Change (TLC) diet recommends:

a. less than 35% of total calories from fat, with less than 10% saturated fat, up to 10% polyunsaturated fat, up to 20% monounsaturated fat, and cholesterol intake less than 300 mg per day; 50-60% of total calories from carbohydrates; and 30-35 grams of fiber per day.

b. less than 35% of total calories from fat, with less than 10% saturated fat, up to 15% polyunsaturated fat, up to 15% monounsaturated fat, and cholesterol intake less than 200 mg per day; 45-50% of total calories from carbohydrates; and 30-35 grams of fiber per day.

c. less than 30% of total calories from fat, with less than 7% saturated fat, less than 10% polyunsaturated fat, 10% monounsaturated fat, and cholesterol intake less than 300 mg per day.; 45% to550% of total calories from carbohydrates; and 25-30 grams of fiber per day.

d. less than 35% of total calories from fat, with less than 7% saturated fat, up to 10% polyunsaturated fat, up to 20% monounsaturated fat, and cholesterol intake less than 200 mg per day; 50-60% of total calories from carbohydrates; and 25 grams of fiber per day.

51. Lifestyle modifications that may help to prevent or manage hypertension include:

a. achieve a healthy body weight; limit alcohol intake to 2 ounces of ethanol for men and 1 ounce for women; increase exercise to a minimum of 60 minutes per day; limit sodium intake to 3,000 mg per day; quit smoking; and reduce saturated fat and cholesterol intake.

b. achieve a healthy body weight; limit alcohol to 1 ounce of ethanol per day for men and 0.5 ounce for women; increase exercise to at least 30 minutes per day; restrict sodium intake to 2,400 mg per day; quit smoking; and reduce saturated fat and cholesterol intake.

c. achieve a healthy body weight; ensure adequate calcium and magnesium intake; eliminate alcohol; restrict sodium to 2,000 mg per day; increase potassium intake to at least 100 mEq per day.

d. achieve a healthy body weight; ensure adequate calcium and magnesium; limit potassium to 90 mEq per day; limit sodium intake to 2,400 mg per day; reduce saturated fat and cholesterol intake; increase exercise to at least 60 minutes per day.

52. The food intake of a patient with chronic obstructive pulmonary disease (COPD) is adversely affected by all of the following EXCEPT:

a. shortness of breath (SOB).

b. problems with food preparation due to increased fatigue.

c. increased oxygen saturation while eating.

d. fluid restriction.

53. An elderly patient with COPD has difficulty maintaining weight, lives alone, and has trouble preparing meals. The correct nutrition interventions include which of the following?

    a.   Instruct the patient to do the following: Eat small, frequent meals and snacks containing nutrient-dense foods and/or supplements; eat slowly, chew thoroughly, and swallow safely to prevent aspiration. Arrange assistance with meal preparation and shopping. Refer to congregate meal program or Meals on Wheels.

    b.   Stock the freezer with easy to prepare frozen dinners and commercially prepared supplements, in case the patient is unable to prepare a meal. Increase the patient's fluid intake to 8-10 cups of fluid per day for adequate hydration. Refer the patient to a home health aide.

    c.   Provide a variety of take-out menus from restaurants that provide free delivery service. Limit meals to 3 per day to lessen meal preparation time. Provide high calorie, high protein snack recipes. Ensure fiber intake is 20-35 grams per day to increase GI motility.

    d.   Enlist help from family and friends for food preparation and clean-up at each mealtime. Encourage the patient to eat the main meal later in the day, after he/she has had a chance to rest. Instruct the patient to lie down immediately after eating to ease digestion.

54. The correct nutritional management for a chronic kidney disease (CKD) patient receiving hemodialysis is:

    a.   30 kcal/kg, 0.8-1.0 g/kg protein; 2-4 g sodium; 2 g potassium, 800-1,200 mg phosphorus; restrict fluid to 1,500 mL per day.

    b.   30-35 kcal/kg, 1.0-1.3 g/kg protein; 3-4 g sodium; unrestricted potassium; restrict phosphorus by limiting dairy to one 8 oz serving or the equivalent per day; unrestricted fluid.

    c.   minimum of 30-35 kcal/kg, 1.2 g/kg of protein; 2-4 g sodium; 2-3 g potassium; restrict phosphorus by limiting dairy to one 8 oz serving or the equivalent per day; fluid intake of 1,000 mL plus the amount of daily urinary output.

    d.   25-30 kcal/kg, 1.5 g/kg of protein; 4 g sodium; 2 g potassium; restrict phosphorus by limiting dairy to one 8 oz serving or the equivalent per day; fluid intake of 1,500 mL plus the amount of daily urinary output.

55. Which vitamin is least likely to be deficient in patients with chronic kidney disease receiving hemodialysis?

    a.   Vitamin D
    b.   Vitamin C
    c.   Vitamin B_6
    d.   Vitamin A

56. Enteral nutrition support for oncology patients is contraindicated for all of the following conditions EXCEPT:

    a.   bowel obstruction.
    b.   nausea and vomiting for 1-2 days following chemotherapy.
    c.   low platelet count.
    d.   severe nausea, vomiting, or diarrhea.

57. Megestrol acetate is for:
    a. nausea and vomiting.
    b. stimulating appetite.
    c. mucositis.
    d. saliva replacement.

58. The nutrition care process is documented on which of the following forms?
    a. ADIME or PGIE
    b. SOAP or PAR
    c. PIE or PAR
    d. PGIE or ADIOP

59. The School Breakfast Program and National School Lunch Programs are administered by the:
    a. USDA.
    b. CDC.
    c. EFNEP.
    d. HHS.

60. The purpose of the Child and Adult Care Food Program is to:
    a. provide guidelines for serving nutritious meals and snacks to daycare programs for children and adults.
    b. provide guidelines for meal patterns and reimbursement for nutritious meals and snacks to child care centers, emergency shelters, and adult day care programs, based on income eligibility.
    c. provide food for meals and snacks for child care centers, emergency shelters, adult day care programs.
    d. provide guidance and resources on appropriate feeding practices throughout the lifecycle for income-eligible participants.

61. The program that provides nutrition education regarding food choices, food safety, budgeting, and gardening to adults and children through many venues is called:
    a. Nutrition Programs for Minority-Serving Institutions.
    b. Eat Better, Move More.
    c. SAP-Ed.
    d. EFNEP.

62. Which of the following is not a nutrition issue that will affect a burn patient's outcome?
    a. Healing of burn injury
    b. Frequently assessing nitrogen balance to indicate anabolism
    c. Providing sufficient calories, so weight loss is less than 10% throughout the burn treatment
    d. Initiating enteral feedings within 4-8 hours of hospitalization with burn injury, and advancing as quickly as possible to optimal nutrient requirements

63. A "house" enteral tube feeding is:
    a. hydrolyzed.
    b. polymeric.
    c. elemental.
    d. modular.

64. The registered dietitian should select an intermittent drip-feeding schedule when a patient needs home enteral nutrition because:

    a. a pump-supported regimen is more cost effective.
    b. it is better tolerated than other types of feeding schedules.
    c. it allows the patient more mobility and time free from the pump.
    d. it reduces aspiration risk.

65. The health care team should conduct all of the following on a patient with an enteral jejunostomy tube EXCEPT:

    a. weight monitoring at least 3 times per week.
    b. monitoring of serum electrolytes and renal function.
    c. monitoring of intake and output records, including bowel movements.
    d. gastric residuals check every 4-6 hours.

66. The stages of change model (precontemplation, contemplation, preparation, action, maintenance, relapse) is also known as the:

    a. cognitive-behavioral model.
    b. transtheoretical model.
    c. interventional model.
    d. motivational model.

67. Which of the following is TRUE regarding implementing dietary change?

    a. Resistance and denial signal noncompliance with the intervention.
    b. A patient progresses through the stages of change in a fluid, forward-moving process.
    c. A patient will only change when he or she is ready.
    d. The RD's counseling style has no impact on a patient in denial, who does not accept the need for change.

68. All of the following techniques are appropriate for the client who resists dietary changes, EXCEPT:

    a. ignoring the individual's perception.
    b. being empathetic to the client's issues.
    c. recognizing cultural factors that create resistance to change.
    d. preventing the client from becoming defensive about his or her lack of motivation.

69. During the first counseling session, the RD uses the intervention model to:

    a. get as much information from the client as quickly as possible.
    b. establish rapport with the client and set the tone for future sessions.
    c. sit across the desk from the client in order to take better notes on what the client is saying.
    d. take charge and recommend dietary changes for immediate implementation.

70. What communication strategies might an RD employ for a client who is not ready to make any dietary changes?

    a. Reflective listening and affirming the client's issues
    b. Summarizing and making an action plan for change
    c. Problem recognition and goal setting
    d. Sending the client away to reflect on the barriers to change and booking a follow-up session for one week later

71. The RD documents all of the following nutrition education items EXCEPT:

   a. the reason for visit and current diagnosis.
   b. short-term and long-term goals, meal planning, and topics covered during education.
   c. RD's thoughts on the client's progress, expected compliance level, and what changes the client has already succeeded in making.
   d. fee schedule and the client's perception of medical care he or she is receiving.

72. The purpose of evidence-based practice is to:

   a. search the internet to find new therapies to treat patients.
   b. use data from cohort studies to change practice.
   c. improve patients' outcomes by incorporating the best research available in new treatments and therapies.
   d. use meta-analyses, review articles, or consensus statements to change the way patient care is provided.

73. Which of the following internet sources is not a primary source for evidenced-based practice?

   a. WebMD
   b. Ovid
   c. PubMed
   d. American Dietetic Association Evidence Analysis Library

74. What kind of research design does the Dietary Approaches to Stop Hypertension Trial (DASH) follow?

   a. Randomized-controlled double blind study
   b. Meta-analysis
   c. Randomized epidemiological study
   d. Cohort study

75. Effective nutrition education materials should have all of the following characteristics EXCEPT:

   a. plain language instead of medical terminology.
   b. grade 12 reading level.
   c. clear, concrete recommendations.
   d. language style that closely reflects that used by the target audience.

76. A requirement for multicultural nutrition counseling includes:

   a. knowledge of different cultures, including eating habits, family traditions, food practices, food preparation, and relevant, specific research.
   b. translation of standard nutrition education materials from English into the appropriate language.
   c. knowledge of appropriate cultural substitutions for Americanized food, to make dietary changes easier.
   d. reluctance to provide personalized nutrition education to a minority culture, if it is not predominant in your area.

77. The body language that indicates a client is open to intervention is characterized by:
a. lowering the eyes, looking away, or lack of eye contact.
b. pupil dilation, nodding head up and down, leaning forward.
c. pursed lips and shaking head from side to side.
d. shrugging shoulders, hanging head down towards chest.

78. To encourage a client in the contemplative stage of change, the RD should:
a. assist the client to make appropriate goals to facilitate change.
b. help the client adjust the changes already made, to further progress.
c. prevent the client from feeling discouraged to help change continue forward.
d. help the client see the advantages and disadvantages of making changes.

79. A hospital menu that rotates daily on a predicted schedule, such as every three days or every week, is called a:
a. limited menu.
b. rotating menu.
c. cycle menu.
d. table d'hôtel menu.

80. The major reason an institution implements a nonselective or preselected menu is most likely:
a. financial.
b. quality.
c. balanced diet.
d. catering for special requests.

81. All of the following characterize the restaurant style of food service EXCEPT:
a. clear, concise, easy to understand menu selections.
b. short explanations about modified diets.
c. room service, where meals ordered by telephone are delivered at the patient's request.
d. less interaction between the patient and food service personnel.

82. If a patient in a long-term care facility requests a write-in or substitution on the menu, the RD's response should be to:
a. immediately disregard the request because it increases food costs.
b. inform the patient that the request was considered but the policy is no substitutions.
c. provide the request or offer another option.
d. inform the patient that at least 48 hours is required to plan for special requests.

83. The first task when planning a cycle menu is to:
a. plan salads, side dishes, and appetizers.
b. plan breakfast entrées.
c. plan starch items and sauces.
d. plan dinner entrées for the whole cycle.

84. The School Meals Initiative for Healthy Children (SMI) requires schools to do all of the following EXCEPT:

    a. decrease the amount of salt and sugar in reimbursed meals.
    b. use one of four menu-planning options, such NuMenus or Enhanced food-based menus.
    c. provide meals consistent with the Dietary Guidelines for Americans.
    d. limit total fat to 40% of total calories for reimbursed meals over the course of a week.

85. What are Standards of Identity?

    a. Any food that crosses US borders must be appropriately labeled.
    b. Food must contain specific ingredients in specified amounts to be labeled with a certain name, such as ice cream.
    c. All foods purchased by food service institutions are labeled with nutrition information and omit any health claims.
    d. A voluntary program that institutions can participate to receive federal funding.

86. Which best qualifies as a Standard of Quality for apple juice?

    a. The quantity of apples used to make apple juice
    b. The type of container used to package the apple juice
    c. The Brix–Acid Ratio
    d. The type of apple used to make apple juice

87. The lowest quality of beef is:

    a. canner.
    b. cutter.
    c. select.
    d. choice.

88. Food production forecasts rely on all of the following EXCEPT:

    a. historical records.
    b. customer demand.
    c. intuition.
    d. menu or event planned.

89. Which of the following determines a registered dietitian's production schedule?

    a. Planning what needs to happen throughout the day, how much food to prepare, yields, employee assignments and general instructions
    b. A timeline of when certain events need to happen throughout the day
    c. Employee work hours, scheduled meals and breaks
    d. Weekly work schedule for the entire food service operation

90. All of the following are advantages of centralized ingredient control EXCEPT:

    a. allowing the cook or chef to focus on production, rather than gathering and measuring ingredients.
    b. cost control.
    c. allowing the chef to improvise recipes to improve customer satisfaction.
    d. allowing partially used packages to be reused and not wasted if the entire package is not required for a recipe.

91. Which food-borne illness incubates 3-5 days and causes diarrhea, nausea, abdominal pain, and headache for 1-4 days?

    a. *Escherichia coli*
    b. *Campylobacter jejuni*
    c. Rotavirus
    d. *Salmonella*

92. Which of the following temperature ranges is considered the danger zone?

    a. 50-150 °F
    b. 40-140 °F
    c. 60-160 °F
    d. 45-145 °F

93. Which form of hepatitis are infected food service workers most likely to transmit?

    a. Hepatitis A
    b. Hepatitis B
    c. Hepatitis C
    d. Hepatitis E

94. The Hazard Analysis Critical Control Point (HACCP) Model is a concept that:

    a. deals with hazardous waste disposal in food service environments.
    b. implements quality control procedures for the prevention of potential microbial or other contaminations.
    c. addresses proper hand washing techniques within the food service environment.
    d. is a mandatory program run by the Food and Drug Administration to promote food safety and to protect the general public.

95. The food service system that partially cooks food, quickly chills it, stores it, and reheats it before client service is considered:

    a. centralized.
    b. decentralized.
    c. commissary.
    d. cook-chill.

96. What is the appropriate temperature for sanitizing utensils and dinnerware in a dishwasher?

    a. 195 °F
    b. 180 °F
    c. 120 °F
    d. 150 °F

97. All of the following precautions should be taken to prevent slips and falls in the work area EXCEPT:

    a. duct tape electrical cords to equipment to prevent tripping.
    b. keep aisles free from obstructions and excessive storage.
    c. clean spills immediately and mark wet areas with appropriate signage.
    d. provide adequate lighting and clean only one side of the work area at a time to allow safe passage through the dry side.

98. A registered dietitian plans to serve employees hamburgers and hotdogs at an outdoor luncheon. The RD must purchase enough 80% lean ground beef to yield 300 hamburgers weighing 3.5 ounces each. How much ground beef is needed?

a. 66 pounds
b. 53 pounds
c. 82 pounds
d. 95 pounds

99. A 4-ounce portion of mashed potatoes is being served on the serving line. What size disher is appropriate?

a. 16
b. 12
c. 10
d. 8

100. All of the following items should be included in a job description EXCEPT:

a. job title.
b. job duties.
c. job specifications.
d. job benefits.

101. The Family Medical Leave Act of 1993 requires:

a. all employers to provide 8 weeks of paid maternity leave coverage to female employees.
b. employers with more than 50 employees must provide all employees up to 10 weeks of unpaid leave with job protection status to care for a newborn, or immediate family member (spouse or child) with a serious health issue, or to deal with a personal health crisis.
c. employers with more than 50 employees must provide all employees who have worked at least 1,250 hours in the previous 12 months up to 12 weeks of unpaid leave with job protection status to care for a newborn, immediate family member (spouse or child) with a serious health issue, or deal with a personal health crisis.
d. all employers must provide up to 12 weeks of unpaid leave to any employee to care for a newborn, ill family member, adopt a child, or to take intermittent time off to receive personal healthcare, such as chemotherapy or physiotherapy.

102. A hospital cook develops unexplained leg pain that prohibits him from standing for long periods. Allowing him to sit while performing his duties is not a reasonable accommodation. Safe cooking and use of food service equipment requires him to stand. Management offers the cook a temporary office assignment, working on production schedules and reviewing standardized recipes. The federal law that protected the cook from job loss is the:

a. Civil Rights Act.
b. Americans with Disabilities Act.
c. Family Medical Leave Act.
d. Worker Adjustment and Retraining Act.

103. During a job interview, a prospective employer asks the interviewee, "Give me an example of a time where you were dealing with a difficult situation and how you resolved this situation." The employer's request is an example of:

    a. structured interviewing.

    b. stress interviewing.

    c. behavioral interviewing.

    d. situational interviewing.

104. Orientation familiarizes new employees with the organization and teaches them how to perform their new job functions. Which of the following is the best orientation process?

    a. The new employee tours the department and reads the Policy & Procedure manual.

    b. A preceptor gives the new employee a tour, explains the job requirements, and directs the initial assignment.

    c. The departmental director welcomes the new employee, gives a tour, completes the paperwork, and tells the new employee to observe another employee who performs the same job.

    d. The RD meets the new employee, explains the purpose of orientation, completes the paperwork, discusses the department's purpose and objectives, introduces other employees, gives a tour of the department and overall facility, reviews Policies & Procedures, explains and demonstrates job duties, and arranges additional observation and training with a preceptor.

105. A performance appraisal is all of the following EXCEPT:

    a. an opportunity for the employee to demand more salary, regardless of the details of the appraisal.

    b. a chance for the employee and the manager to discuss job performance.

    c. a method of identifying goals and objectives in the coming year for the employee.

    d. a chance to list strengths and weakness and to identify strategies for meeting unmet job performance standards.

106. What is an advantage of scheduling personnel for a cook-chill food service?

    a. Fewer FTE's are required overall because it is a simpler type of food service system to operate.

    b. Most production and inventory FTEs are scheduled during off-peak hours Monday to Friday, leaving a few FTE's for meal-times and weekends.

    c. Most FTEs are scheduled in the early morning hours or weekends.

    d. Scheduling is closely related to the tray line operation, and this type of system has peak and trough employee activities.

107. A food service manager is often responsible for scheduling the:

    a. production schedule.

    b. master schedule.

    c. shift schedule.

    d. all of the above.

108. All of the following are reasons for an employee to join a union EXCEPT:

a. dissatisfaction with management rules and policies.
b. compensation and benefit packages.
c. worries about job security.
d. unions require all employees to join if the workplace is an open shop.

109. All of the following are components of a total budget EXCEPT the:

a. operating budget.
b. labor budget.
c. master budget.
d. capital budget.

110. An effective manager possesses which of the following skills?

a. Interpersonal, technical, conceptual
b. Interpersonal, supervisory, technical
c. Conceptual, analytical, contractual
d. Technical, behavioral, conceptual

111. Classical management theory is the belief that:

a. improving employee relations, such as conflict resolution, group dynamics, and increasing motivation, is the way to increase productivity
b. the means to increasing productivity and efficiency is through process improvement
c. computer models and mathematical equations can improve productivity
d. management has the final say in all matters and employees must learn to accept this

112. The management theory that incorporates Maslow's Hierarchy of Needs is which of the following?

a. Classical
b. TQM
c. Behavioral
d. Integration

113. All of the following violate the Dietetics Code of Ethics EXCEPT:

a. the RD in private practice actively promotes specialized vitamins and minerals and benefits financially from sales, but does not tell the client of her personal involvement with the products.
b. the RD food service manager in a hospital kitchen depends on painkillers to control pain from a running injury and takes them while on the job.
c. the clinical RD exhibits symptoms of bipolar disorder while at work and various coworkers complain. The RD receives psychiatric treatment but later refuses medication due to its side-effects.
d. a clinical RD dates another RD, who is the assistant manager in the food production area.

114. Which best describes the difference between a nutritionist and a registered dietitian?

 a. State licensure laws define the term nutritionist and the scope varies greatly. Only candidates who pass the dietetic registration examination can legally use the title Registered Dietitian, and they must remain in good standing with the Commission on Accreditation for Dietetics Education.

 b. A registered dietitian holds a master's degree and passed a national registration examination. A nutritionist completed a 4-year Bachelor of Nutrition degree but did not take the registration examination.

 c. A registered dietitian completed the minimum requirements set forth by the Commission on Accreditation for Dietetics Education and passed the registration examination. A nutritionist provides any type of nutrition advice or counseling and is accredited by the National Association of Nutritionists.

 d. A nutritionist has a master's or doctoral degree in a nutrition-related field but is not a registered dietitian. A registered dietitian completed the minimum requirements set forth by the Commission on Accreditation for Dietetics Education and successfully completed the registration examination.

115. Total Quality Management includes all of the following maxims EXCEPT:

 a. processes are changed, not people.
 b. the customer is the main focus.
 c. employees must follow their job descriptions with minimal variation from procedure.
 d. a team approach is the optimal way to improve quality and ensure long-term change.

116. What is the purpose of Press Ganey Associates, Inc.?

 a. Consulting
 b. Benchmarking
 c. Job redesign
 d. Quality Assurance

117. The process the Joint Commission uses to survey healthcare organizations is called a:

 a. tracer process.
 b. performance measurement process.
 c. self–study process.
 d. patient-centered process.

118. Which documentation is prohibited according to the Joint Commission's Do Not Use List?

 a. 90 mL of sterile water
 b. 10.0 mg of Lipitor QD
 c. 10 mg morphine sulfate
 d. 400 international units of vitamin D

119. All of the following are valid ways to reduce food costs EXCEPT:

 a. set up security measures in production areas.
 b. use seasonal items for special menus or meals whenever possible.
 c. change menu prices in the employee cafeteria all at once, rather than one at a time.
 d. frequently compare competitive vendors' prices to ensure you receive the lowest prices.

120. A registered dietitian is a food service manager. Two of the workers do not work well together. The RD frequently hears them bicker and yell at each other and calls a conflict resolution meeting with both of them. How should the RD initiate conflict resolution?

- a. Ask each worker for his/her side of the story. Assess the situation. Gently point out the person who needs to make changes.
- b. Ask each worker to relate his/her version of events calmly. Restate the issue in your own words. Get additional information. Mutually agree on what the problem actually is. Brainstorm possible resolutions. Negotiate an acceptable resolution for both of them.
- c. Tell the two employees their behavior is inappropriate. Listen to both sides. Determine if there is an easy fix to the problem. Warn the employees that they must both resolve the issue or they will be disciplined.
- d. Allow the senior employee to tell his/her side of the story first. Reprimand the employee who is at fault. Offer anger management classes to both employees.

121. A customer evaluating a meal's quality is least likely to consider:

- a. taste, appearance, and portion size.
- b. service and preparation method.
- c. quality of ingredients.
- d. popularity of the item in the cafeteria.

122. A food manager is least likely to evaluate customer satisfaction in the hospital cafeteria by:

- a. entrance interviews.
- b. customer surveys.
- c. talking to customers at the end of their meals.
- d. customer comment cards.

123. All of the following factors influence an employee's job satisfaction EXCEPT:

- a. personality and values.
- b. work environment and the job itself.
- c. gender.
- d. social influences, such as co-workers and culture.

124. The type of pricing strategy that a food service manager uses to price menu items by adding a markup value is known as:

- a. prime cost.
- b. factor pricing.
- c. actual cost.
- d. combination pricing.

125. The leadership style of a Clinical Nutrition Manager who manages a staff of clinical dietitians strictly "by the book", with a clear division between the manager and the clinical staff, is known as:

- a. participative.
- b. authoritarian.
- c. delegative.
- d. diplomatic.

Answer Key and Explanations

1. C: Maltose. A monosaccharide is the smallest carbohydrate unit with the formula $(CH_2O)_n$. Fructose is a sugar found in fruit and is the sweetest of all monosaccharides. Galactose is not found freely in foods but is derived from the hydrolysis of the milk sugar lactose during digestion. Glucose is the primary monosaccharide used for energy. Glucose is generally part of a disaccharide linked to fructose in the form of sucrose or linked to lactose in the form of galactose. When glucose is linked with another glucose molecule, it forms maltose and is considered a disaccharide.

2. B: The liver stores approximately 100 grams of glycogen. Glycogen is a form of short-term carbohydrate storage for the body. It is not a long-term energy source. Approximately 100 grams of glycogen is stored in the liver, which when catabolized provides approximately 400 kcals. About 300-400 g of glycogen is stored in the skeletal muscles, which yields less than 1,600 kcal. Glycogen is not stored in the heart muscle. The glycogen stored in the liver provides energy anywhere in the body, whereas the glycogen stored in the skeletal muscles provides energy only to skeletal muscle cells. The amount of stored glycogen is sufficient to sustain a 70 kg male for approximately 1 day.

3. D: Glucocorticoids, such as cortisol, stimulate glycolysis to increase blood glucose levels. Blood glucose levels are influenced by hormones, drugs, and vagus nerve activity. The islets of Langerhans in the pancreas produce insulin when the patient feeds and glucagon when the patient fasts. In the postprandial period, β (Beta) cells release insulin to normalize blood glucose levels. In the fasting state, α (Alpha) cells release glucagon to stimulate glycogenolysis, which is glycogen breakdown. Epinephrine and norepinephrine increase glucose levels during stress by promoting catabolism of muscle cells for glycogen and adipose cells for triglycerides. Glucocorticoids increase blood glucose levels by stimulating gluconeogenesis, not glycolysis. Glycolysis is the breakdown of glucose. Gluconeogenesis is glucose formation, which occurs mainly in the liver. Glycolysis and gluconeogenesis do not occur at the same time.

4. C: Provide a source of eicosapentaenoic (EPA) and docosahexaenoic (DHA) essential fatty acids. Fat plays a very important role in the body. It provides a concentrated energy, at 9 kcal/g, whereas protein and carbohydrate only provide 4 kcal/gg. Structural fat pads cushion and protect the body from injury, especially bones and internal organs. Fat provides a source of essential fatty acids, which the body does not manufacture, but must obtain from seeds, oils, cold-water fish, or supplements. The three essential fatty acids (EFAs) are arachnoidic, linoleic, and linolenic. EFAs are important for blood clotting and brain development. Eicosapentaenoic (EPA) and docosahexaenoic (DHA) derive from α-linolenic acid, but are not themselves essential fatty acids. Fats are also required for the absorption of the fat-soluble vitamins A, D, E, and K.

5. D: Tyrosine, glycine, alanine. Amino acids are the building blocks of protein. There are 20 amino in total. Nine amino acids are essential and cannot be manufactured by the body: Isoleucine, leucine, lysine, methionine, phenylalanine, threonine, tryptophan, valine, and histidine. Often, adults can synthesize enough histidine, but infants and children cannot. Essential amino acids must be obtained from food. The best sources of essential amino acids are animal products, such as meat, poultry, fish, dairy, and eggs. A diet containing 10-12% of calories from protein should meet essential amino acid requirements. The non-essential amino acids are arginine, alanine, asparagine, aspartic acid, cysteine, glutamine, glutamic acid, glycine, proline, serine, and tyrosine.

6. A: Excessive protein intake is difficult to achieve and, therefore, is not a danger. The majority of Americans consume protein in excess of requirements. Many people consume at least

24

twice as much as they need. Some excess protein becomes a calorie source or converts to fat. Studies demonstrated an increase in calcium excretion related to an increase in protein intake, especially animal protein, due to acidified blood. As the digestive system breaks down large amounts of protein, the bones release calcium to neutralize the blood. Acidified blood leads to osteoporosis in predisposed people. Normally functioning kidneys excrete nitrogenous wastes, including urea derived from the breakdown of protein. Athletes often consume more protein in the false hope that it will build bigger muscles. There is no benefit to massive protein intake. Actual muscle development results from exercise, weight training, and proper nutrition.

7. B: 66 grams. In the described meal, the protein content is 66 grams, as follows: Fish 42 grams; pasta 6 grams; broccoli 4 grams; whole wheat bread 2 grams; milk 8 grams; and angel cake 3 grams.

The American Dietetic Association's book, Choose Your Foods: Exchange Lists Diabetes, offers a quick way to calculate the macronutrient content of many foods:

- Meats and meat substitutes contain 7 grams protein per ounce
- Starches contain 3 grams of protein per serving
- Vegetables contain 2 grams of protein per serving
- Milk contains 8 grams of protein per 8 ounce serving
- There is no significant protein in fruit

Check the serving size, as portion sizes vary between food items.

8. A: Loss of somatic stores. Kwashiorkor is malnutrition from lack of amino acids. It usually affects weaned children between 12 months and 3 years old in Third World countries with famine, drought, political unrest, or traditional eating habits. The victim's diet is protein-deprived. Most calories are derived from a restricted carbohydrate source, such as corn or sugar-water. Kwashiorkor is uncommon in the United States, where it usually appears only in severely abused children and neglected nursing home residents. The main characteristics include preservation of somatic or fat stores and loss of visceral protein stores. The signs and symptoms of kwashiorkor are: A large, protruding belly; significant edema; changes in hair and skin pigment; skin rash; fatigue; irritability; diarrhea; and decreased immune function. Victims never reach their height potential.

9. C: Severe malnutrition, with loss of subcutaneous fat and depletion of muscle mass, followed by a breakdown in lean body mass. Marasmus is severe malnutrition from lack of calories. It usually affects infants 6-18 months old when their mothers' breast milk fails and they contract chronic diarrhea from polluted water. It can also affect children with metabolic disorders or malabsorption. Marasmus is characterized by a decrease in somatic and subcutaneous stores, preservation of visceral protein stores, depletion of lean body mass, pronounced weight loss (emaciation) to 20% of normal for a given height, large head, loose skin, intellectual disability, depression, and failure to thrive. By contrast, kwashiorkor affects children 1-3 years old with depleted visceral protein stores, but somatic and subcutaneous fat stores are preserved. Mixed malnutrition (marasmic kwashiorkor) means both calories and protein are deficient and features of both conditions are present.

10. C: The most active form of Vitamin D is 25-hydroxycholecalciferol and occurs after hydroxylation in the liver. Vitamin D is obtained through fortified dietary sources and sunlight exposure. Vitamin D is activated by two hydroxylations:

- The first occurs in the liver and produces 25-hydroxycholecalciferol, the main circulating form of vitamin
- The second hydroxylation occurs in the kidney where 1, 25-dihydroxyvitamin D is produced, the most active form of vitamin D (also called calcitriol)

Vitamin D has many functions, but mainly it promotes calcium and phosphorus homeostasis. Vitamin D also plays a role in skin, muscle and nerve function, cell differentiation, and immune function.

11. D: Baked potato. Niacin is found in many foods, including chicken, turkey, lean meats, and fish. Niacin is one of four vitamins added to enriched grain products (flour, cereals, and breads). Beans, seeds, legumes (peanuts and lentils) are good sources of niacin. Milk, coffee, and tea provide some niacin. Vegetables are not a significant source of niacin, except for mushrooms. Most people get plenty of niacin from their diets and do not require a supplement. Large doses of niacin are sometimes used to treat hypercholesterolemia under medical supervision. Significant side-effects may occur, such as severe flushing or itching skin, and liver damage.

12. B: Consuming a high-protein meal promotes zinc absorption through the formation of zinc-amino acid chelates, a more easily absorbed form of zinc. A high protein meal does promote zinc absorption. Zinc is absorbed at the brush border of the small intestine. The human body typically absorbs only 20-40% of zinc ingested. Pregnancy and lactation actually increase zinc absorption. Zinc must be protein-bound to be absorbed. Therefore, the protein in the meal helps to form zinc-amino acid chelates that enhance absorption. Phytates interfere with the absorption of zinc; however, it appears that tannins do not. Soy protein improves zinc absorption.

13. A: An infant loses weight initially after birth, regains it by Day 10, doubles birth weight by 6 months, triples birth weight and doubles length by his/her first birthday. An infant's birth weight is determined by gestational age, mother's weight before pregnancy, and weight gain during the gestation period. It is normal for a newborn infant to lose up to 10% of its birth weight in the first few days of life. This is not cause for concern, unless the infant continues to lose weight after the tenth day of life. Most infants double their birth weight by 6 months and triple it by their first birthday. Length usually doubles within the first year. Weight gain and growth are influenced by both nutrition and genetics. The growth percentiles determined at birth are not usually the best indicators of overall growth. The majority of infants settle into their own growth curve somewhere between 3 and 6 months of age.

14. C: Up to 40% reduction in resting metabolic rate, due to reduced lean body mass, since muscle is the most metabolically active tissue. The aging process essentially begins after the age of 30. The body has reached physiological maturity and the rate of catabolism is greater than the rate of anabolism. The aging process is influenced by genetics, socioeconomic status, overall health, activity level, and lifestyle. Lean body mass is lost at a rate of 2-3% per decade and it is often replaced with fat. Lean body mass is the most metabolically active tissue, so its loss reduces the resting metabolic rate by 15-20% over the course of a lifetime. Other physiological changes include nephrons loss in the kidneys and achlorhydria, which is reduced stomach acid affecting the absorption of Vitamin B_{12} and subsequent pernicious anemia in elders.

15. D: Iron. A child grows rapidly from the ages of 1-3 years. Some children are at risk for malnutrition because they are very fussy eaters, or are not offered appropriate foods to meet nutritional needs, or have a reduced appetite. The need for protein decreases as the child gets older. Most children consume more protein than is needed by the body. It is easy to meet the requirements for Vitamin C with a daily serving of juice. Calcium deficiency occurs if a child does not consume any sources of calcium. Iron deficiency is most likely to occur following the rapid growth of infancy, as there is an increase in hemoglobin. Many children's diets lack iron and its absorption rate can be decreased by many factors.

16. B: The purpose of a nutrition screen is to identify people with malnutrition or who are high-risk for developing malnutrition. Nutrition screening is a part of the nutrition assessment process. Screening can be completed by a registered dietitian, dietetic technician, physician, nurse, or an appropriately trained delegate. The main purpose of the nutrition screen is to identify malnourished individuals or those who are at risk for developing malnutrition. Screening enables the practitioner to identify those individuals who are in need of a full nutrition assessment by the registered dietitian. Although the elderly population does greatly benefit from frequent nutrition screening, the tool is useful for all age groups. The major components of a nutritional screen are: Measuring height and weight; determining weight changes; and checking laboratory data. However, the information gathered for the screen varies, depending on its setting, the target population, and its identified goals.

17. D: American Medical Association. The Nutrition Screening Initiative of 1990 was a partnership between the American Academy of Family Physicians, the American Dietetic Association, and the National Council on Aging. The partners wanted to develop a tool to improve nutritional care for the elderly. They developed a simple checklist screening tool and two levels for further evaluation, which the patient can complete independently, or a medical professional can administer. Many community agencies administer the screen to populations they serve.

18. C: Disease, Eating Poorly, Tooth Loss/Mouth Pain, Economic Hardship, Reduced Social Contact, Multiple Medicines, Involuntary Weight Loss/Gain, Needs Assistance in Self-Care, Elder Years Above Age 80. The acronym DETERMINE was developed as part of a nutrition checklist to help remind patients and caregivers about the warning signs and risk factors in the elderly population for developing malnutrition. The letters stand for Disease, Eating Poorly, Tooth Loss/Mouth Pain, Economic Hardship, Reduced Social Contact, Multiple Medicines, Involuntary Weight Loss/Gain, Needs Assistance in Self-Care, Elder Years Above Age 80. The checklist asks questions that delineate warnings, such as, "I have an illness or condition that made me change the kind and/or amount of food I eat". The evaluator tallies the patient's responses to determine the overall level of nutritional risk, which varies from low, to moderate, to high risk.

19. D: Supplemental Nutrition Assistance Program. The Head Start Program requires that a child's medical needs are up-to-date and his/her nutritional needs are addressed within 90 days of enrollment. The Special Supplemental Nutrition Program for Women, Infants, and Children (WIC) documents nutritional risk when the participant is certified. The Farmer's Market Nutrition Program is a part of the Special Supplemental Nutrition Program for Women, Infants, and Children program in 45 states. Participants currently enrolled in the WIC program are eligible for the Farmer's Market by using separate coupons issued along with the participants' regular WIC benefits. The Supplemental Nutrition Assistance Program (SNAP, formerly known as the Food Stamp Program) is based mainly on income level. Nutrition screening in not part of the SNAP process.

20. A: A validated nutrition screening and assessment tool to identify the presence or risk of malnutrition in patients 65 and older. The Mini Nutritional Assessment (MNA) is a tool developed for people over the age of 65 to screen for malnutrition. The MNA is an easy, validated tool that provides talking points for practitioners to obtain additional necessary information, when indicated. MNA helps to identify malnutrition in the elderly, to enable earlier nutrition intervention, and to prevent worsening of the condition. The MNA form requires the patient's: Age, gender, weight; height; food intake; weight loss; mobility level; presence of stress; change in diseases status; changes in mental capacity; living situation; prescription drug use; and skin condition.

21. D: A federal program that combines an interview with a physical exam to assess the general health and nutritional status of participants of any age living in the United States. The National Health and Nutrition Examination Survey (NHANES) is a federal program that surveys the health and nutrition status of both children and adults in the United States. The program obtains information through an interview process. The interviewer gathers data about the participants' demographics, socioeconomic status, diet, and health. The interview is followed by a physical examination that includes laboratory tests and medical, dental, and anthropometric measurements. The NHANES survey helps to establish national standards for health issues, such as blood pressure and extremes of weight. The data obtained is available for epidemiological research throughout the world. Past surveys produced data that helped researchers develop growth charts for infants and children, policies benchmarking blood lead levels, and increased public awareness about diseases, such as diabetes.

22. C: The program originated in the 1960s through the Surgeon General's Report on Health Promotion and Disease Prevention. Healthy People 2030 is an extension of a health prevention program that originated in 1979 through the Surgeon General's Report on Health Promotion and Disease Prevention. The program's main goals are to increase the overall quality of life and the number of years spent in good health, and to eliminate disparities in health between different parts of the population. There are 62 topic areas divided across five categories: Health conditions, health behaviors, populations, settings and systems, and social determinants of health. 355 total measurable objectives were created that can be used by states, local communities, and various organizations and institutions. Some of the focus areas include cancer, obesity, diabetes, health communication, oral health, and food safety.

23. C: Food/nutrition-related history; biochemical data and medical tests; anthropometric measurements; nutrition-focused physical findings; and client history. Nutrition assessment is the first step in the Nutrition Care Process. The purpose of an assessment is to gather and explain all the appropriate data needed to determine any nutrition-related issues, why they occurred, and their level of importance. Data for the Nutrition Assessment piece of the Nutrition Care Process can be obtained from a variety of places, including conversation with the patient, medical records, or from consulting another healthcare practitioner. The data is organized into 5 categories: Food/nutrition related history, biochemical data and medical tests, anthropometric measurements, nutrition-focused physical findings, and client history.

24. A: Nutrition-focused Etiology. The second step of the Nutrition Care Process is Nutrition Diagnosis. The goal of a Nutrition Diagnosis is to recognize and delineate a particular nutrition issue that can be treated with nutrition intervention, with positive results. A registered dietitian (RD) completes a nutrition diagnosis. The RD utilizes the data gathered in step 1 of the Nutrition Care

Process to identify and assign a specific nutrition diagnosis. Nutrition diagnoses are organized into 3 different categories:

1. Intake, which compares the amount of food or specific nutrient consumed to what the estimated or actual requirements are
2. Clinical, which links nutrition issues to a particular medical disorder
3. Behavioral/environmental which looks at the specific nutrition knowledge, belief, and access to nutrition and food safety

25. B: Evaluating the etiology, determining if the best "root cause" has been identified, and determining if the signs and symptoms can at least be improved with nutrition intervention. The RD requires critical thinking skills to perform nutrition care, particularly when assigning a nutrition diagnosis. The RD documents the nutrition diagnosis with a PES statement (Problem-Etiology-Signs/symptoms). The nutrition diagnosis the RD selects should be the most important that requires the most immediate attention. It is not necessarily the diagnosis that will see the fastest results. The diagnosis the RD selects should be most related to the RD's role in the Nutrition Care Process and be specific enough to measure concrete improvement. Clinical judgment is still important. However, nutrition intervention must be measured and documented. At the very least, the RD's involvement should help to minimize any symptoms that are present.

26. A: The physician determines the medical diagnosis, while the RD determines the nutrition diagnosis. Part of the reason for introducing the Nutrition Care Process was to standardize nutrition care in a systematic way. Using standardized terminology is a step in this direction. Medical diagnoses are made by the physician, whereas nutrition diagnoses are determined by the RD. Both diagnoses can be mutually exclusive. Nutrition diagnoses can also be different, based on individual patients with the same diagnosis. For instance, two different patients have heart disease, but one is overweight and the other is not. The RD must address the overweight patient's weight reduction in the nutrition diagnosis as excessive energy intake.

27. C: Excessive energy intake related to frequent consumption of fast food, as evidenced by BMI and diet history. In this scenario, we do not know what additional exercise the patient gets besides walking to restaurants. His is 20 pounds overweight and has been diagnosed with heart disease, which we know is a modifiable risk factor. We do not know the period in which he gained weight. The best PES would be defining the problem as excessive energy intake. The etiology of the problem would be increased consumption of fast foods. The signs and symptoms would be the BMI of 26 and his diet history.

28. D: Altered nutrition-related lab values, physical inactivity, or overweight/obesity. The nutrition diagnosis is a problem the RD labels, addresses, improves, and resolves. Diabetes mellitus is a medical diagnosis but not a nutrition diagnosis. Instead of using diabetes mellitus, it would be appropriate to use the nutrition diagnosis of altered nutrition-related lab values. In this case, fasting blood glucose falls under behavioral-environmental. From the information provided, we do not know what this woman's diet history is. We are then unable to assign a nutrition diagnosis related to her carbohydrate intake or energy intake, until we obtain this information. We do know that her physical activity is inadequate, which also falls under behavioral-environmental. We do know from her BMI of 28 that she is overweight and this is a clinical finding.

29. B: Excessive smoking. There are many potential nutrition diagnoses for this patient. The best choices are inadequate energy intake because of the weight loss, swallowing difficulty causing the patient to alter the consistency of his diet, and involuntary weight loss. Excessive smoking is not a nutrition diagnosis, but it likely does influence his medical diagnosis. Another potential nutrition diagnosis would be altered nutrition-related laboratory value because his serum albumin level was low. There are no right or wrong nutrition diagnoses but they must be well thought out and prioritized in order of importance. The primary nutrition diagnosis must be something the RD can influence and potentially resolve.

30. D: Both retrospective data collection, such as food frequency or 24-hour recall, and prospective data collection, such as food record or food diary. To obtain information for a dietary history, the RD collects retrospective data, prospective data, or a combination of both. Retrospective data is information recalled from the patient or client's memory. Retrospective data collection includes food frequency questionnaires or 24-hour recall. The concerns about retrospective data collection include its validity, reliability, memory issues, and inaccurate reporting. Prospective data collection is information recorded around the time the food is eaten. Examples of prospective data collection are calorie count or nutrient intake records, food records, and food diaries.

31. A: Pregnant women. Nitrogen balance is a way to assess overall protein status. To calculate nitrogen balance, determine how much protein is ingested, how much nitrogen is excreted, and how much nitrogen disappears through insensible losses, such as sweating and skin sloughing. The equation is: Nitrogen balance = Nitrogen intake (grams/24 hours) – (Urinary nitrogen [grams/24 hours] + 2 grams/24 hours

Normal, healthy adults have a zero-nitrogen balance. A positive nitrogen balance is seen in pregnant women, growing children, and patients rebounding from an injury or sickness. Negative nitrogen balance occurs in starvation.

32. B: C-reactive protein. Inflammatory stress can be caused by acute trauma or injury. During the stress response, acute-phase proteins are released or utilized to meet the crisis. Examples of positive acute-phase proteins are C-reactive protein and fibrinogen. The level of acute-phase proteins during the immediate inflammatory stage reflects the degree of injury. Examples of negative acute-phase proteins include albumin, retinol-binding protein, and transferrin. The levels of negative acute-phase protein vary, based on the rate of increased catabolism or a decrease in synthesis.

33. C: Measuring serum albumin is a valuable tool in assessing short-term changes in protein status. Serum albumin is a negative acute-phase reactant with a half-life of 20 days. This means albumin is very slow to show changes in protein status. It is a better indicator of long-term changes in protein status, or to measure maintenance of albumin in a stable, long-term patient. Since albumin is an acute phase reactant, levels decrease during infection, trauma, inflammation, and acute injury. Prealbumin is a better marker of short- term changes in protein status. The half-life of prealbumin is 2 days. It is also known as thyroxin-binding prealbumin (TTHY).

34. B: A patient with low homocysteine has an increased risk of developing CVD.
Homocysteine levels are linked to the development of cardiovascular disease as an independent risk factor. Elevated homocysteine levels, even in the upper normal range, correlate with an increased CVD risk. Homocysteine levels are affected by diet. Folate, Vitamin B_6 and Vitamin B_{12} supplements will help to lower homocysteine levels. Clinical trials are being conducted to determine if lowering homocysteine levels actually has a positive impact on the reduction of CVD. It currently appears that those patients who would benefit most from lowered homocysteine levels are those with a history of CVD, but without other major risk factors, such as smoking, hypertension or high serum cholesterol.

35. A: Central obesity (waist circumference greater than 40 inches for men, 35 for women), fasting glucose levels greater than or equal to 100 mg/dL, blood pressure greater than 130/85 mmHg. Metabolic syndrome means the patient has a group of risk factors related to overweight or obesity, lack of exercise, and predisposing genetic factors, which increases his/her risk for developing coronary heart disease. At least three of the following risk factors are required for a diagnosis of metabolic syndrome: Central or abdominal obesity with a waist circumference of 40 inches for men and 35 inches for women; fasting serum triglyceride levels greater than or equal to 150 mg/dL; an HDL level less than 40 mg/dL for men and 50 mg/dL for women; fasting glucose level greater than or equal to 100 mg/dL; or a blood pressure reading greater than or equal to 130/85 mmHg.

36. A: Small frequent meals with high protein, moderately fatty foods; limited concentrated sweets; and drinking liquids separately from meals. Dumping syndrome may occur following GI surgery, due to changes in gastric emptying in response to a meal. The goal of medical nutrition therapy is to prevent dumping symptoms from occurring by manipulating the diet and timing of meals:

- Small, frequent meals spread throughout the day
- Moderate fat intake of 35-45% of total calories to slow transit time.
- Protein intake increased to 20% of total calories
- Complex carbohydrate intake
- Fluids consumed separately from meals, as too many fluids may increase transit time
- Lactose avoidance

Fiber does help to slow transit time; however, fibrous foods may cause bowel obstruction.

37. B: Nutrition is a major issue for both Crohn's disease and ulcerative colitis patients; however, malnutrition is likely to be more of a lifelong concern for patients with ulcerative colitis. Crohn's disease and ulcerative colitis are the two main forms of IBD. The age of onset is usually between the ages of 15 and 30, and sometimes between 50 and 60. Both diseases have similar symptoms, including diarrhea, weight loss, fever, anemia, and food intolerances. Both types of IBD are likely to cause malnutrition. However, patients with Crohn's disease are more likely to have prolonged malnutrition over the course of a lifetime, due to management issues. Crohn's disease can occur in segments anywhere within the GI tract but is most likely to occur in the distal ileum and colon. Patients with Crohn's disease often require surgical treatment but surgery does not cure the disease. Many Crohn's patients develop additional complications, such as short bowel syndrome. Ulcerative colitis occurs only in the colon.

38. C: Anthropometric data, including information on weight changes and visual assessment. Nutritional assessment of patients with end stage liver disease is often difficult because many test parameters are adversely affected:

- BUN is useless because nitrogen builds up in the form of ammonia, so BUN cannot be interpreted in the usual way
- Creatinine height index is compromised by decreased liver function (synthesis of creatine to creatinine occurs in the liver)
- Serum albumin and other visceral protein levels are unreliable, as the liver synthesizes visceral proteins
- Anthropometrics are unreliable, due to fluid retention and use of diuretics

Instead, take a weight history and perform a visual assessment. Look for muscle wasting and the presence of fat stores. Added to the overall subjective global assessment, these two parameters are most useful.

39. B: In uncomplicated hepatitis or cirrhosis without encephalopathy, protein requirements are 1.0-1.2 grams per kilogram of dry weight to promote nitrogen balance. Protein requirements in chronic liver disease remain controversial. The European Society of Parenteral and Enteral Nutrition (ESPEN) recommends giving patients with compensated liver disease 1.0-1.3 grams of protein per kilogram, including patients with chronic cirrhosis without encephalopathy. Measure the patient's dry weight to calculate his/her protein requirements, as many patients with liver disease have ascites. For patients with acute encephalopathy, the generally accepted practice is to restrict protein intake to 0.6-0.8 grams per kilogram, but only during the acute phase. After the encephalopathy clears, restore protein intake to 1.0-1.2 grams per kilogram. Patients with compensated liver disease and malnutrition may require up to 2 grams of protein per kilogram, providing their renal function is normal.

40. A: Provide IV fluids for hydration until the patient is pain-free and nausea and vomiting have resolved. Initiate a clear liquid diet and gradually advance to a soft, low-fat diet based on patient tolerance. Acute pancreatitis is sudden inflammation of the pancreas, causing intense abdominal pain, nausea, and vomiting. Symptoms worsen when the patient consumes food, due to pancreatic stimulation. Treatment for acute pancreatitis is:

1. Allow the pancreas to rest by keeping the patient NPO (nothing by mouth).
2. Start IV fluids for hydration.
3. If the acute illness does not resolve promptly, start enteral feedings for patients who require nutrition support. Use a chemically-defined formula fed into the jejunum for the least pancreatic stimulation.
4. Initiate parenteral nutrition after 5-7 days if the patient remains severely ill.
5. When the patient can tolerate oral feedings, initiate a clear liquid diet and progress to a soft, low-fat diet. Small, frequent meals are often better tolerated than three large meals. Added pancreatic enzymes are typically not required for acute pancreatitis patients.

41. B: Meal planning that incorporates the individual's usual eating and exercise habits, followed by development of an insulin regimen. Presently, the insulin options available to help the patient get diabetes under control are fast-acting and slow-acting injections and pumps. The RD's main priority for treating an insulin-dependent Type 1 diabetic is to determine the patient's usual eating and exercise patterns. Try to maintain consistent meal timing and carbohydrate distribution. Assigning an inflexible meal and snack pattern is unrealistic and encourages non-compliance. Many diabetics learn how to manage flexible insulin regimens based on the amount of carbohydrate consumed at a given meal. Take into account the patient's established physical activity routine. Advise the patient who does not engage in regular exercise to incorporate physical activity into his/her lifestyle gradually. Adjust the diabetes regimen accordingly.

42. D: Modify fat intake to help prevent the development of cardiovascular disease and improve lipid panel; modify protein intake to help prevent the development of nephropathy and other kidney-related complications.

The main goals of medical nutrition therapy for diabetes are essentially the same for all patients, regardless of age:

- Keep blood glucose, lipid levels, and blood pressure within recommended ranges to prevent or delay potential complications of diabetes
- Encourage weight loss for patients who are overweight or obese
- Adjust nutrient intake as needed, if complications are present, but otherwise encourage healthy dietary choices and exercise

Do not modify the protein intake of diabetics who have normal kidney function. Some diabetics may have protein requirements slightly above the RDA. There is no evidence to prove that higher protein intake causes diabetes-related nephropathy.

43. C: Alcohol is an energy source that is not converted to glucose, unlike food. Alcohol inhibits gluconeogenesis, which can lead to hypoglycemia if you drink alcohol on an empty stomach. Explain alcohol's effect on metabolism to the diabetic, so he/she can make an informed decision about drinking alcohol. Alcohol is an energy source and adds calories to the diet. It is not metabolized into glucose, as food is. Alcohol inhibits gluconeogenesis, which in turn prevents glucose from entering the bloodstream in response to insulin secretion, leading to low blood glucose. The low glucose response is potentiated if the patient drinks alcohol on an empty stomach. Exercise also lowers blood glucose levels, so drinking alcohol after exercise and taking insulin or oral hypoglycemics greatly increases the risk of hypoglycemia. It also makes recovering from a low blood sugar reaction more difficult until the alcohol is metabolized completely. Limit alcohol consumption to one drink per day for women and two for men.

44. D: The onset of action is 2-4 hours, peak action is 6-10 hours, and the duration is 10-16 hours. The different types of insulin currently available are injections and pumps of rapid and short-acting, intermediate-acting, long-acting, and premixed. Oral sprays and skin patches are now in development. NPH and Lente are examples of intermediate-acting insulin. Give intermediate-acting insulin twice per day, once before breakfast and the other later at dinner or bedtime. The onset of action is approximately 2-4 hours. The peak action occurs around 6-10 hours. The duration of intermediate insulin is 10-16 hours. Check the effects of intermediate insulin within 8-12 hours, to ensure the patient's blood glucose is in the proper range. Short-acting insulin begins to work within 1 hour. Its peak is within 2-3 hours. Its duration is 3-6 hours. Long-acting insulin begins to work within 6-10 hours. It peaks around 10-16 hours. Its duration is 18-24 hours.

45. B: Consume only sugar-free fluids to prevent hyperglycemia from an excessive sugar intake. Emphasize the importance of sick day management to your Type 1 diabetic patients. Failure to follow these guidelines could cause diabetic ketoacidosis (DKA):

- Always take insulin as prescribed during an illness. Sometimes insulin requirements increase due to infection, fever, or stress.
- Test blood glucose levels, urine, or blood ketones at least four times throughout the day. The presence of ketones along with a blood glucose level greater than 240 mg/dL signals that DKA is developing.
- If regular foods are intolerable, substitute soft foods or liquids containing carbohydrates. Sugar-free or low carbohydrate foods are not indicated.

33

- Consume at least 50 grams of carbohydrate every 3-4 hours and maintain adequate hydration.
- If the illness continues beyond 24 hours, contact a physician.

46. A: If the patient's blood glucose level is less than 70 mg/dL, give 4 ounces of juice or 1 tablespoon of sugar. Recheck the patient's blood glucose level in 15 minutes. If the level remains less than 70 mg/dL, give another 15 grams of carbohydrate. A blood glucose level less than 70 mg/dL is hypoglycemia and requires immediate attention. Use the "Rule of 15" to remember the treatment guidelines: If the blood glucose level is low, give 15 grams of carbohydrate. For example, 4 ounces of juice or other sugary beverage, 3-4 glucose tablets, 6-8 Lifesavers, or 1 tablespoon of sugar or honey. Recheck the blood glucose level again in 15 minutes and if it is still low, give another 15 grams of carbohydrate. Recheck the blood glucose level again in 15 minutes. Blood glucose levels may drop again within an hour. Therefore, if a meal or substantial snack is not planned within an hour, give another 15 grams of carbohydrate.

47. B: The LDL cholesterol level is the primary marker, followed by the presence of coronary heart disease, and risk factors (smoking, hypertension, HDL levels less than 40 mg/dL, age greater than 45, or significant family history). The ATP III guidelines are part of the National Cholesterol Education Program (NCEP). Use the patient's LDL cholesterol level as the primary marker for initiating therapy. A level less than 100 mg/dL is optimal; 100-129 is near optimal; 130-159 is borderline high; 160-189 is high; greater than 190 is very high and dangerous. ATP III also uses total cholesterol and HDL levels as secondary markers. Evaluate the presence of coronary heart disease or other types of atherosclerotic diseases, such as carotid artery disease or peripheral arterial disease. Next, assess the number of modifiable and non-modifiable risk factors: Smoking; HDL level less than 40 mg/dL; hypertension; family history of early heart disease, such as a male first degree relative diagnosed prior to age 55 or a female first degree relative diagnosed earlier than age 65; patient's age (men older than 45 or women older than 55). Categorize the patient's overall risk. Base initial treatment on LDL cholesterol levels.

48. C: A child must have a nutritious diet containing a variety of food groups; total fat intake of 25-35% of total calories for children older than 4; mostly monounsaturated or polyunsaturated fat; five fruits and vegetables per day; whole grain products whenever possible; low fat or fat-free dairy products for children older than 2; and at least one hour of exercise most days of the week. The American Heart Association recommends heart-healthy choices parents can make for their children. Start healthy choices in infancy. Children 2-3 years old should have a fat intake that is 30-35% of total calories. After age 4, reduce total fat intake to 25-35% of total calories. Offer a variety of foods, starting as early as possible. Restrict juice intake but encourage intake of whole fruits and vegetables. Offer whole grains and low fat or fat-free dairy products for children older than 2. Provide enough calories for normal growth and development, without overfeeding. Weight loss is not necessarily the goal for most children who are overweight. Adjust their calorie intake to slow the rate of weight gain and increase their amount of physical activity, with a goal of 60 minutes most days of the week.

49. B: HDL cholesterol, dietary modifications, and LDL cholesterol. Reducing or eliminating modifiable risk factors has a direct impact on lowering cardiovascular events. Modifiable risk factors include: Quitting smoking; lowering LDL cholesterol; lowering blood pressure; making diet dietary changes to reduce fat and cholesterol; effective diabetes control; exercise; increasing HDL cholesterol; weight loss; and lowering triglyceride levels. Modifiable risk factors are measurable. Document patient outcomes to measure progress. Other modifiable risk factors that may or may not influence CVD risk are reducing oxidative stress levels, lowering homocysteine, and reducing alcohol intake. Non-modifiable risk factors are age, gender, family history, and the mere presence of diabetes.

50. D: Less than 35% of total calories from fat, with less than 7% saturated fat, up to 10% polyunsaturated fat, up to 20% monounsaturated fat, and cholesterol intake less than 200 mg per day; 50-60% of total calories from carbohydrates; and 25 grams of fiber per day. The Therapeutic Lifestyle Change (TLC) diet is part of the National Cholesterol Education Program (NCEP). The TLC diet replaces the former American Heart Association Step 1 and 2 diets. The recommendations for the TLC diet are as follows: Less than 7% of total calories from saturated fat; 25-35% of total calories from fat; less than 200 mg per day of cholesterol; up to 10% of total calories from polyunsaturated fat; up to 20% of total calories from monounsaturated fat; 50-60% of total calories from carbohydrates; 25 grams of fiber per day; 15% of total calories from protein. Weight loss or maintenance is important, as is regular and consistent physical activity.

51. B: Achieve a healthy body weight; limit alcohol to 1 ounce of ethanol per day for men and 0.5 ounce for women; increase exercise to at least 30 minutes per day; restrict sodium intake to 2,400 mg per day; quit smoking; and reduce saturated fat and cholesterol intake.

Lifestyle modifications have a huge impact on preventing and managing hypertension. Changing four modifiable risk factors makes the biggest impact on blood pressure:

6. Achieve and maintain a healthy body weight
7. Limit alcohol intake to 1 ounce of ethanol (24 ounces of beer, 10 ounces of wine, or 2 ounces of hard liquor) for men and 0.5 ounce of ethanol for women
8. Restrict sodium intake to 2,400 mg per day
9. Increase physical activity to at least 30-45 minutes per day for the majority of the week

Other lifestyle changes that improve blood pressure modestly are: Increasing calcium and magnesium intake; receiving at least 90 mEq of potassium per day; lowering saturated fat and cholesterol; and quitting tobacco use.

52. C: Increased oxygen saturation while eating. A COPD patient has difficulty consuming enough food, due to shortness of breath. Dyspnea decreases oxygen saturation. Advise your COPD patient to use oxygen while eating to help alleviate dyspnea. Often, liquids are easier for COPD patients to consume, rather than chewing and swallowing foods. Consider this before you decide to restrict fluids for a COPD patient. Many individuals with COPD have difficulty preparing meals, due to fatigue from oxygen deprivation. Anorexia or poor appetite is related many chronic diseases, including COPD. The COPD patient's metabolism changes and energy requirements are often increased, due to the increased work of breathing and the type of treatments required (e.g., physiotherapy and steroid medications).

53. A: Instruct the patient to do the following: Eat small, frequent meals and snacks containing nutrient-dense foods and/or supplements; eat slowly, chew thoroughly, and swallow safely to prevent aspiration. Arrange assistance with meal preparation and shopping. Refer to congregate meal program or Meals on Wheels. Tell the elderly patient with COPD who lives alone to consume small, frequent meals and snacks, to emphasize nutrient-dense foods, and eat the main meal early in the day. Foods should be relatively easy to chew to help the COPD patient swallow safely and reduce the risk of aspiration. Arrange a visiting homemaker to assist this patient with shopping and meal preparation. Book the patient for a congregate meal program, if possible. If the patient finds congregate dining too stressful, arrange Meals on Wheels delivery. Stocking the freezer with frozen dinners is not a good option because it increases sodium

35

intake. Commercially prepared supplements (e.g., Ensure) provide calories and protein, but they should not be used consistently as meal replacements. If the patient is using diuretics, discuss the amount of fluid needed each day with the physician.

54. C: Minimum 30-35 kcal/kg, 1.2 g/kg of protein; 2-4 g sodium; 2-3 g potassium; restrict phosphorus by limiting dairy to one 8 oz serving or the equivalent per day; fluid intake of 1,000 mL plus the amount of daily urinary output. An ESRD patient receiving hemodialysis treatments does require nutritional management. Energy intake should be 30-35 kcal/kg but can vary, based on the patient's overall clinical condition. Protein requirements are 1.2 grams/kg or higher depending on protein status. Sodium restriction is required for blood pressure management and fluid status. When the patient's kidney function has deteriorated enough to require hemodialysis, a potassium restriction of 2-3 grams per day is usually sufficient to maintain serum potassium in the normal range, but adjust potassium as needed. Phosphorus restriction of 800-1,200 mg per day is usually required, even if the patient already uses phosphorus binders. Limit fluids to the amount of urinary output plus 1,000 ml. Monitor weight gain between treatments. Weight gain from dry weight should be less than 3 kg.

55. D: Vitamin A. Vitamin deficiency is a concern for patients with chronic kidney disease because their diets are restricted for fruits, vegetables, and dairy products. Adding dialysis to the equation increases their risk for Vitamin C and Vitamin B deficiencies, as these vitamins are lost through dialysis. Rarely do patients with ESRD develop Vitamin A deficiency. The amount of retinol-binding protein is usually elevated in the blood of patients with CKD, indicating potential toxicity. Supplementation of Vitamin A is not recommended. Vitamin D is converted to its active form in the kidney. With kidney failure, this process cannot occur. Provide the active form of Vitamin D as calcitriol to prevent deficiency.

56. B: Nausea and vomiting for 1-2 days following chemotherapy. Enteral nutrition may be appropriate for cancer patients who are not expected to regain improved oral nutrition within five to seven days after chemotherapy. If the patient's GI tract is fully functional, then choose enteral nutrition in the form of tube feedings. If the patient is only symptomatic for 1-2 days following chemotherapy, but is then able to maintain reasonable oral intake, tube feedings are not indicated. Definite contraindications to tube feeding include bowel obstruction, severe nausea or vomiting, and diarrhea. Oncology patients with low platelet counts should not receive tube feedings, as the risk of bleeding is increased. Other contraindications include overall low white or red counts, as these may signify infection.

57. B: Stimulating appetite. Megestrol acetate is commonly used to stimulate appetite in oncology and other disease states that produce anorexia, such as HIV. It is synthetic form of progesterone. Do not use megestrol as a preventative measure. It helps to increase weight gain by increasing the appetite, and thus food intake. Known side-effects of megestrol acetate include endocrine suppression, edema of the hands and feet, thrombophlebitis, and changes in blood glucose levels. Therefore, monitor fluid balance, hormone levels, and signs of clotting closely. Other medications used to stimulate appetite include dronabinol and dexamethasone.

58. A: ADIME or PGIE. Documentation of the nutrition care process may include one of six formats using acronyms. It helps to incorporate the PES statements, interventions, monitoring and evaluation as a part of the nutrition care process. The first is called ADIME and stands for Assessment, Diagnosis or PES statement, Intervention, Monitoring and Evaluation. The second is PGIE, which stands for Problem or diagnosis, Goal, Intervention, and Evaluation. Next is SOAP, which stands for Subjective, Objective, Assessment/diagnosis, and Plan. DAR stands for Data/diagnosis, Action/nutrient prescription/ nutrition intervention and Response. This can also be documented as DAR-O if it includes Output. Lastly, PIE is another format that stands for Problem/diagnosis, Intervention, and Evaluation.

59. A: USDA. The School Breakfast Program and National School Lunch Program are administered by the United States Department of Agriculture (USDA). The CDC stands for Centers for Disease Control. EFNEP stands for Expanded Food and Nutrition Education Program. HHS stands for Department of Health and Human Services. HHS is responsible for protecting the health of all Americans and for providing essential human services, such as the Headstart Program or improving child and maternal health. The USDA administers other types of programs, such as WIC, SNAP (food stamps), Child and Adult Care Food Program, and the Special Milk Program. HHS is also is involved in other nutrition initiatives, such as the website nutrition.gov for consumer nutrition information, and meat and poultry hotlines for consumer food safety information.

60. B: Provide guidelines for meal patterns and reimbursement for nutritious meals and snacks to child care centers, emergency shelters, and adult day care programs, based on income eligibility. The Child and Adult Care Food Program is a program administered by the USDA. It is geared to low-income individuals and families. The program provides meal-planning guidelines for all ages, including infants up to the elderly. The location of the program may include childcare centers, after school programs for at-risk children, group daycare homes, emergency shelters and adult daycare centers. Meal reimbursement is provided according to guidelines set forth by the agency. Eligibility is based on income levels between 130-185% of the federal poverty level. The federal program provides funds to state agencies to distribute.

61. D: EFNEP. The Expanded Food and Nutrition Education Program (EFNEP) was designed to help individuals and families of limited resources learn about nutrition-based behaviors that can improve their diets and overall wellbeing. EFNEP instructors teach adults about shopping and budgeting strategies, cooking techniques, food safety, and sanitation. EFNEP is a very "hands-on" program to enhance kinesthetic learning. For children and adolescents, the program may be part of community centers, 4-H groups, after school programs, or daycare centers. Children may learn about gardening, food preparation, food safety, and how nutrition and health are related.

62. B: Frequently assessing nitrogen balance to indicate anabolism. Nutrition support is a cornerstone in the treatment of burn injuries. Actual healing is the best outcome one can observe and is directly related to nutrition. Accurately assessing nitrogen balance for a burn patient is difficult, due to potential nitrogen losses through large open wounds, but it can be calculated. It is better to assess wound healing and the progress of the grafts as an outcome measure. Maintain the patient's weight within 10% of normal to promote overall healing. Very early enteral nutrition helps decrease the catabolic rate and improves the overall outcome for the burn patient. Lower catabolism decreases the overall length of hospital stay. Enteral nutrition stimulates immune function and protects against GI bleeds.

63. B: Polymeric. A polymeric formulation is typically known as a "house" formulation. Polymeric formulae contain an intact protein source, such as caseinate, or soy protein isolate. Polymeric formulae are isotonic, can be initiated at full strength, and are usually tolerated very well. The caloric density of a polymeric formula is 1.0-1.2 calorie/mL. Polymeric formulae can also contain fiber to aid bowel function. Hydrolyzed formulae contain dipeptides as the protein source. Elemental formulae contain free amino acids. A modular product means single nutrients were added in-house to change the overall composition of a commercially-prepared product.

64. C: It allows the patient more mobility and time free from the pump. Intermittent feeding schedules are often the schedule of choice for patients who require tube feedings at home and are able to ambulate fairly well. Plan an intermittent schedule with or without the use of a feeding pump. The schedule is generally four to six feedings per day of a specific volume administered over a period of 30-60 minutes. Many patients who are alert, ambulatory, and able to perform self-care tolerate an intermittent schedule very well. Patients who are at risk for aspiration should not receive an intermittent feeding schedule. Intermittent feedings used without a pump can be more cost-effective than a continuous feeding schedule.

65. D: Gastric residuals check every 4-6 hours. Any patient receiving enteral nutrition must have a planned monitoring schedule, including a patient with a nasogastric tube, gastric tube, or jejunostomy tube. The doctor orders lab tests according to the institution's specific protocols. Monitor the patient's laboratory results for serum electrolytes, renal function, glucose, calcium, phosphorus, magnesium, albumin, and nitrogen balance. The nurse weighs the patient at least three times per week and the RD should check the results. Work with the nurse to monitor the patient's intake and output (urine and stool) and ensure the patient receives adequate nutrition and hydration. For nasogastric and gastric tube patients, monitor gastric residuals as a precaution. The validity of monitoring residuals remains unclear, as there may be 150 mL or more in the stomach at any given time, due to gastric juices. Do not check feeding tubes in the jejunum because there is no reservoir, as in gastric feedings.

66. B: Transtheoretical model. The stages of change model (transtheoretical model) describes six alterations a patient experiences when trying to adjust to a change. The RD assesses which stage of change the patient is in during a counseling session. In the precontemplation stage, the patient has not yet thought about making any changes. In the contemplation stage, the patient begins to think of reasons why he should or should not make changes. In the preparation stage, the patient may be ready to move ahead and requires assistance finding a strategy that will work. In the action phase, the patient begins to make the necessary changes. In the maintenance stage, the patient must continue to follow through with positive behaviors. Lastly, in the relapse stage, the patient must begin the change process again after a failure, to achieve the action phase.

67. C: A patient will only change when he or she is ready. When an RD tries to help a patient make dietary changes, the RD must remember the patient will only make a change when he or she is ready to do so. The patient who is in the action or maintenance stage of change is ready to adjust. A patient who resists or is in denial may eventually make dietary changes, but at the moment, he or she is not yet ready. The rate of progress through the stages of change is an individual journey. The patient may move forward or backward at any time. People do not move along in a predetermined sequence. It is important for the RD to determine which stage of change the patient is in to tailor counseling efforts appropriately. The RD's counseling style, personality, and what he or she addresses motivate the patient to make a change.

68. A: Ignore the individual's perception. An effective counselor recognizes certain behaviors on the dietitian's part influence client behavior. The RD should always try to be empathetic when a client expresses concerns about implementing change. Empathy is an important tool for effecting change. Cultural issues have a significant impact on change and the RD should be aware of these. For example, Koreans may automatically agree with everything someone in charge says, even though they may have no intention of implementing any of the suggestions. The RD must not place the client in a position where he/she becomes defensive. The RD tries to offer support and encouragement. An impasse means a change in counseling strategy is in order. The RD should not ignore a client's perceptions, though. Identify any perception that may interfere with change and explore it.

69. B: Establish rapport with the client and set the tone for future sessions. Establishing a rapport with a client is essential to the counseling process. Establish rapport by asking a few general questions about the client's personal life. Try to find a common ground. Examples of this may be mutual enjoyment of a certain sport or type of animal. Use your first session for information gathering. Do not rush due to time constraints or money. Use the corner of a desk for note taking, but do not use it as a barrier between you and the client. Seating yourself beside the client is less intimidating than sitting across from the client, behind a desk. Never try to take charge of the session immediately, as this does not invite effective change. First, complete the assessment piece and identify the patient's stage of readiness. Give positive reinforcement for changes the client has already made or is already performing correctly.

70. A: Reflective listening and affirming the client's issues. Effective communication skills help a client address reasons why change will be difficult. Reflective listening means listening closely to what a client is saying, then rephrasing as a short statement to show you comprehend the issue. Affirmation means demonstrating your appreciation of a client's attempts at changing behavior. Let the client know you understand the issues and that it is normal to have roadblocks to progress. Summarize what your client says. Identify and label the conflicting issues. Ask open-ended questions that allow your client to expand on his or her thoughts, rather than provide a yes or no answer. Do not immediately set goals or an action plan for a client who is not yet ready to change.

71. D: Fee schedule and the client's perception of medical care he or she is receiving. Do not include the client's fee schedule when documenting patient education, as this is not pertinent information. Remember that the patient's chart is a subpoenable document that a judge may review. It is illegal to erase or paint correction fluid a charting error. Draw a single line through the error in dark blue or black ink. Write the correction above the error, initial and date it. You must document the reason for the patient's visit, his or her current diagnosis, any relevant lab results, medications, and the name of the physician who referred the patient to you. Briefly outline the History, the nutrition problem list, and the care provided by the physician, including goals set and expected level of compliance. Document all topics you address during the session, dietary changes successfully implemented, and a follow-up plan.

72. C: Improve patients' outcomes by incorporating the best research available in new treatments and therapies. Evidence-based practice incorporates the best available research with clinical expertise, and an individual patient's beliefs and situation into a comprehensive treatment plan. The gold standard for research is randomized, controlled trials that are well designed. Cohort studies, meta-analyses, review articles and consensus statements are useful supplements, but are not the primary mode of obtaining information. Beware of Internet misinformation; ensure any websites you rely on end in .EDU, .GOV, or .ORG. Utilizing evidence-based practice is a way for clinicians to remain well informed and to change practice when new treatments or therapies are available. National accreditation standards require dietitians to follow best practice guidelines and evidence-based practice.

73. A: WebMD. Many legitimate internet sources for evidence-based research exist, such as the US National Library of Medicine's PubMed and Ovid, and the Centers for Disease Control. Do not use WebMD as a primary information source because it is geared to patients, rather than professionals. It may contain valuable information for consumers, but is too simplistic for healthcare professionals. Use websites ending in .ORG, .EDU, or .GOV for reliable research. The American Dietetic Association's Evidence Analysis Library is a database that sorts through important and relevant nutrition research. Two other appropriate databases are SCHARR (School of Health and Related Research) and EMBASE (the Excerpta Medical Database). Individual resources for medical professionals include UpToDate, Harrison's Principles of Internal Medicine, and Clinical Evidence.

74. C: Randomized epidemiological study. The DASH Trial was a multi-center, randomized, controlled feeding study that examined three different meal patterns over an 8-week period:

- A control group who ate a diet low in fruits and vegetables
- A test group with a diet high in fruits and vegetables
- A test group with a diet high in fruits and vegetables and low in saturated and total fat

DASH used a large study sample and four collection centers to gather the research information. Study participants were given the food they were to consume, and were randomly assigned into one of the groups.

A randomized, controlled, double-blind study means neither the study participants nor the researcher knows who receives the test substance and who does not, so the results are more accurate. A meta-analysis is a statistical approach to reviewing similar literature. The researcher combines the data to determine statistically significant results. A cohort study observes a particular group (similar in age, race, or another significant indicator) over a long period. A cohort study is relevant for one group, not able to be extrapolated to the general population.

75. B: Grade 12 reading level. It is difficult for the RD to develop written patient education material because the education levels of the whole population varies greatly and English is not the first language for many readers. Write nutrition information at a Grade 5 or 6 level. Follow plain language guidelines from the federal government at http://www.plainlanguage.gov/. Deliver the message in the easiest, simplest way possible. Omit medical terminology if possible. If medical jargon is required, explain the term within the text and in a glossary. Write in a conversational style mimics the way your target audience speaks. Use short sentences and paragraphs. Use a 12-point font in a standard typeface (Arial, Times New Roman, or Verdana). Leave white space and ragged right margins to make reading easier for the elderly and learning disabled. Make clear, concise recommendations with common examples. Place a relevant illustration above an explanation.

76. A: Knowledge of different cultures, including eating habits, family traditions, food practices, food preparation, and relevant, specific research. The RD must counsel clients who are not of his/her culture, race, religion, ethnicity, or socioeconomic status. Multicultural nutrition counseling skills are a job requirement for RDs in the United States. The RD's professional Code of Ethics requires the RD to give the highest of quality nutrition counseling available to all patients. This requires that the RD research the specific cultures that they frequently contact. The RD should also learn their food practices, eating habits, family traditions, food preparation and food storage practices. Get a translator to tailor existing English material to the target population. Do not merely translate material verbatim. Remember than many immigrants in the United States continue to eat their native foods. The RD should ask their supervisor to schedule cultural sensitivity training for staff as well.

77. B: Pupil dilation, nodding head up and down, leaning forward. Reading body language is an important skill an RD uses to assess a client's stage of readiness. Assume your client is open to nutrition intervention if his/her pupils are slightly dilated, signifying interest, and he/she leans forward and nods his/her head up and down in agreement. Look for direct eye contact, smiling, positive behavior, or a change in position from sitting back to leaning forward. Lowered eyes or looking away can mean fixation on something else or avoidance of the situation in an American-born client, but in other cultures direct eye contact is considered rude and challenging. Pursed lips may mean the client is stressed, angry, or taking psychiatric drugs. Shaking the head from side to side may signal disagreement. Shrugging the shoulders can mean indifference or uncertainty. If the client hangs his/her head down, this may mean sadness, anxiety, or lordosis from a deteriorating spine.

78. D: Help the client see the advantages and disadvantages of making changes. A client in the contemplative stage of change remains indifferent or uncertain about making dietary changes. The contemplative client thinks about making a change but may find a reason to opt out of it. The RD's job in the contemplative stage is to help the client see why making changes would benefit him/her. Do not begin goal setting, as the client will likely tune out. Help your client to adjust before proceeding to the action stage. Prevent your client from feeling discouraged. Move forward by making positive changes until the maintenance stage.

79. C: Cycle menu. A cycle menu rotates every day on a predetermined schedule such as every week or two weeks. Due to shorter patient stays in hospitals, some food services reduce their cycle to a three-day rotation. At the end of the cycle, the menu repeats. The purpose of a cycle menu is to help the patient or visitor feel that meals are not repetitive. Cycle menus save time because when the cycle is planned once, menu planning and recipes are complete. The menu planner should take seasonal produce into account. The purchaser knows what foods need to be ordered and available for each day of the cycle, which helps control costs. Training of production and preparation personnel is tailored to the cycle.

80. A: Financial. Healthcare institutions implement nonselective or preselected menus for financial benefit. Dietary staff or the ward clerk visits the patient on admission to obtain food preferences and potential allergies. A computer-generated menu is released for the patient each day, based on the master menu that has already been planned. Labor costs are reduced because the patient is not seen by staff every day for menu selection. Fewer personnel are required for food production and the tray line. Nonselective and preselective menus also decrease food costs up to 20% because of less waste and leftovers. Other benefits of preselection are limiting the menu to a few main items provides a balanced diet and allows excellent preparation of specialties.

81. D: Less interaction between the patient and food service personnel. A restaurant style menu in a hospital increases patient satisfaction and menu variety. A room service option may be available, where the patient phones the kitchen to order a meal at will and has it delivered in a timely manner. A restaurant style menu should be clear, concise, and easy to read and understand. Remember that patients are incapacitated or medicated and may have difficulty focusing their eyes. Offer explanations about diet modifications and basic nutrition advice on the menu. Restaurant style menus are not designed for less interaction with food service personnel. Frequent, positive interaction with food service personnel improves patient satisfaction.

82. C: Provide the request or offer another option. Many institutions, especially long-term care facilities, try to provide increased choices for patients or may liberalize diet modifications. Still, patients may have special requests known as substitutions or write-ins. The Centers for Medicare and Medicaid Services (CMS) require that substitutions should be honored in long-term care facilities. Other types of institutions should either provide the request or find another option that is amenable to the patient. Exotic requests may be difficult or impossible to provide. Most are reasonable, do not take much effort to provide, and increase patient satisfaction. Keep a list of potential write-in requests available in the kitchen to ease the process.

83. D: Plan dinner entrées for the whole cycle. The RD must the dinner entrées first when preparing a cycle menu because dinner is the most expensive meal of the day. All entrées must be balanced, varied, and within budget. Consider alternatives for vegetarian clients or those with cultural restrictions (e.g., Kosher for Jews and Halal for Muslims). Secondly, plan the lunch entrées.

Thirdly, plan the starch choices, followed by salads, side dishes, and appetizers. Plan desserts after the balanced dinners and lunches. Finally, plan the breakfast meal. Perform a final review to ensure the overall menu is balanced and meets any required government regulations and accreditation standards. Review the results of the last accreditation survey for your department to pinpoint the weak areas in your kitchen.

84. D: Limit total fat to 40% of total calories for reimbursed meals over the course of a week.
The School Meals Initiative for Healthy Children (SMI) requires schools to implement guidelines within their food service operations to help improve the health of our children through improved nutrition. Meal planning must be consistent with the Dietary Guidelines for Americans. Four choices are available for assistance with menu planning: NuMenus, Assisted NuMenus, Enhanced Food-Based, and Traditional Food-Based. Some of these require computer resources, which may not be an option for all schools. Other guidelines include reducing the amount of salt and sugar found in meals, and to limit fat to 30% of total calories and saturated fat to 10% of total calories for meals that are reimbursable. Increase the fruit and vegetable choices for your students. Provide one-third of the Recommended Dietary Allowances for protein, calcium, iron, and Vitamins A and C for lunch and one-quarter of these for breakfast.

85. B: Food must contain specific ingredients in specified amounts to be labeled with a certain name, such as ice cream. Standards of Identity is part of the Food Drug and Cosmetic Act of 1938, which requires any food item that is shipped across state lines to be labeled in a way that accurately reflects what is in the package. If a product is given a certain name, then it must contain specific ingredients in a certain percentage to qualify for that name. For example, ice cream is a frozen product that must contain no less than 10% milk fat and 20% total milk solids by weight. If it does not meet these standards, it is labeled with another name, such as reduced-fat, light or fat-free ice cream. Standards of Identity help the consumer identify what a food product actually contains.

86. C: The Brix–Acid Ratio. Standard of Quality is part of the Food, Drug and Cosmetic Act of 1938, which specifies certain factors that must be present in a food product and objective measures to determine compliance. Standard of Quality helps the consumer to determine the value or use of a product. For example, quality standards can describe: How much water is added to canned foods; how fibrous green beans should be; or what mixed nuts are called, based on the composition of nuts. The quality of apple juice includes its color, clarity, defects, flavor, acidity, and aroma. All of these factors are graded to determine if the juice is of A, B, or Std. quality. The Brix-Acid ratio explains the amount of soluble solid in the juice (the number of grams of acid per 100 grams of concentrated juice).

87. A: Canner. Inspectors grade beef according to its tenderness, amount of marbling, and flavor. Only certain types of cattle are eligible to quality for each grade. For example, meat obtained from mature cows cannot be prime grade. Only meat must from steers or heifers of a certain age and specification qualify for prime grade. The eight grades of meat are: Prime, Choice, Select, Standard, Commercial, Utility, Cutter and Canner. The lowest three grades of beef are rarely used in commercial food service establishments. Manufacturers use cheap cuts for highly processed products, such as hot dogs or canned corned beef.

88. B: Customer demand. The RD reads the requirements of the planned event, reviews historical data, intuits what food customers may demand, and determines a menu. The RD must keep careful production records that document differing factors that influence production, such as: Day of the week; special conditions, such as a holiday or weather events; type of food prepared; quantity prepared; and quantity served. Customer satisfaction is most likely to result when customers get what they ordered and expected, but this is not the deciding factor in a forecast. During a disaster, war, pandemic, or drought, giving adequate nutrition to the greatest number of people is more important than customer satisfaction. Forecasting models are available to reduce the RD's forecasting time. However, they require computer resources, so are usually an option for food service managers only, rather than junior dietitians.

89. A: Planning what needs to happen throughout the day, how much food to prepare, yields, employee assignments and general instructions. The production schedule, also known as the production worksheet, is the main tool for controlling what goes on within the kitchen on a given day. The production schedule sets menu preparation in motion. Always base production of the planned menu on standardized recipes. Individualize the production schedule for your institution. Include on the production schedule for each day: The number of customers; type of weather; pertinent special events; individual employee assignments; timeline for delivery, storage, food preparation and clean-up; any substitutions; actual yield; notations on under-production or over-production; specialized instructions. You require all of this information for accurate future forecasting.

90. C: Allowing the chef to improvise recipes to improve customer satisfaction. Centralized ingredient control is an important part of a cost-effective food service operation. Use an Ingredient Room to distribute menu items or recipe components, as it helps control costs. Do not require the chef or cook to perform tasks for which he/she is overqualified, such as storage and cleaning, as it raises costs. Delegate scut work to less qualified staff and allow the chef to focus on food preparation and presentation. Store incompletely used packages for another recipe. Prevent the chef or cook from trying to use up the product at one session, thus changing the standardized recipe you developed for Quality Control. Centralized ingredient control allows you to combine the same task for different recipes, such chopping green peppers for pizza and chili.

91. B: *Campylobacter jejuni* has long affected animals and has now crossed over to humans. It is a severe form of gastroenteritis, featuring diarrhea, fever, nausea, stomachache, and headache. The incubation period is 3-5 days. Symptoms last up to 4 days. Campylobacter jejuni is can be found in raw vegetables, chicken, pork, beef, and lamb. Avoid cross-contamination by careful hand washing. Use separate cutting boards and utensils for cutting meats and vegetables. Cook foods thoroughly. Wash raw foods extremely well before consuming and peel them, if possible, to prevent transmission.

92. B: 40-140° F. The danger zone is the temperature range at which bacteria are likely to grow and cause illness if consumed. The danger zone is 40-140 °F. Bacteria multiply very quickly within this temperature range. Keep serving dishes hot with warmers or the range. Do not leave serving dishes at room temperature for more than 2 hours. Cool cooked foods as quickly as possible. Refrigerate all cooked foods within 2 hours. Do not thaw frozen on the counter at room temperature. Thaw frozen foods in the refrigerator, instead. Reheat foods to an internal temperature greater than 145 °F. Follow the USDA guidelines for cooking meats, chicken, and egg products to the proper internal temperature.

93. A: Hepatitis A. Hepatitis is inflammation the liver caused by one of five viruses. The five known types of hepatitis are A, B, C, D, and E. Usually, Hepatitis A spreads through contaminated food or water. Sometimes, it spreads through oral/anal contact with an infected person. Hepatitis A spreads quickly in food service establishments when an infected employee does not wash his/her hands thoroughly after using the bathroom. The incubation period for Hepatitis A is 28 days. Hepatitis A is transmissible for 2 weeks before these symptoms appear: Fever; anorexia; nausea; abdominal pain; and jaundice. Instruct any food service worker infected with Hepatitis A to stay out of work at least 2 weeks after symptoms appear. Most people who get Hepatitis A recover completely. Hepatitis E spreads through infected water. Hepatitis B, C, and D spread through infected blood or sexual contact with an infected person. Twinrix vaccine prevents the spread of Hepatitis A and B only and Employee Health offers it free to hospital workers.

94. B: Implements quality control procedures for the prevention of potential microbial or other contaminations. The Hazard Analysis Critical Control Point (HACCP) Model is a plan to prevent microbial contamination through Quality Control. HACCP is voluntary program sponsored by the Food and Drug Administration that aims to protect public health through food sanitation and safety. Its seven guiding principles are:

1. Analyze hazards
2. Identify critical control points (CCPs, a certain step in the preparation of a recipe or in the cooling process)
3. Institute preventive measures
4. Develop procedures to monitor CCPs
5. Develop a corrective action plan and rewrite procedures to fix the faulty CCPs
6. Keep records diligently
7. Base the QA program on appropriate research and studies

95. D: Cook-chill. A cook-chill system is part of a ready prepared food service system. A cook-chill system means the food is partially cooked, then quickly chilled, and stored until it is needed. Food is then reheated and served immediately. Hospitals frequently use the cook-chill method using microwaves, convection ovens, or specially made rethermalization carts. Commissary service is a centralized facility that ships food to several distant facilities, where preparation is finished and food is served. Centralized service means patient trays are prepared in the main kitchen and production area, then delivered and served to patients. Decentralized service means food is sent to galley kitchens for heating and tray assembly, and then food is served to the patients in designated areas, rather than a dining hall.

96. B: 180 °F. The two types of dishwasher machines available to food service establishments are high temperature machines and chemical sanitizing machines. A human dishwasher is also required to scrape plates, load and unload, troubleshoot, inspect the results, discard rejects, and store clean dishes. The wash cycle's temperature varies between different dishwasher machines. However, the Food and Drug Administration's (FDA) Food Code requires the final rinse temperature must be 180 °F for proper sanitization. A 180 °F rinse is hot enough to kill most fungi, bacteria, and viruses but does not kill spores. The plate and cutlery are clean but not sterile. A rinse temperature above 195 °F vaporizes water and does not flush any debris stuck on the plates and utensils.

97. A: Duct tape electrical cords to equipment to prevent tripping. Slips and falls can cause very serious injuries to employees and customers. The RD is responsible for ensuring all kitchen staff take proper precautions to prevent injuries. The Occupational Safety and Health Administration (OSHA) has many regulations in place to help maintain a safe environment, online at http://www.osha.gov/. Ideally, plug electrical equipment into floor or ceiling outlets to prevent tripping on the cord. If you require a wall plug temporarily, tape the cord into place. This should not be a permanent solution. Keep aisles and hallways free from obstructions and clutter. Ensure the kitchen and dining room are well lit. Inspect carpets to insure they are appropriately installed, so no bunching occurs. Remove worn carpeting. Remember that tile floors are more hygienic. Report spills and wet areas to Housekeeping immediately for clean-up. Mark wet area with warning signs. Provide staff with ladders or step stools, instead of chairs or boxes, so they can reach items on high shelves safely.

98. C: 82 pounds. Yield is how much product is produced at the end of the production process. As purchased (AP) is the amount of product you need to buy to achieve the yield. Edible portion (EP) is how much product is available after the production process, including peeling and cooking. In the above example, if the final yield is 300 hamburgers at 3.5 ounces after cooking, a total of 1,050 ounces of 80% ground beef is required (after cooking weight). One pound of 80% lean ground beef yields 0.8 pounds of edible portion. The AP will be 1,312.5 ounces (1,050 ounces ÷ 0.8). Divide by 16 to convert to pounds. Your result should equal 82 pounds of 80% lean ground beef.

99. D: 8. A disher is also known as a scoop size. A disher helps with portion control. Portion control is very important, both for controlling food costs and for promoting customer satisfaction. Food service managers and employees must understand the need to control portions, and must remember the quantity each disher, ladle, and pan will yield. A number 8 disher is approximately 8 tablespoons, or ½ cup, and has an approximate weight of 4-5 ounces. Dishers are typically even-numbered, ranging from 6 down to 100. A size 6 measures 2/3 cup. A size 100 measures 2 teaspoons.

100. D: Job benefits. A job description is a document that describes the various tasks, requirements, working conditions, necessary tools and equipment, and responsibilities involved in a certain job. A job description has three main sections: Job title, job identification, and job duties. Job title is important because it allows the employee to know exactly where he/she fits into the organization (org chart). Job identification identifies to whom the employee will report. Job duties list the job functions and responsibilities in order of their importance. Some job descriptions include an additional job specifications section, which lists the necessary education, registration, skills, and training, required to perform the job legally.

101. C: Employers with more than 50 employees must provide all employees who have worked at least 1,250 hours in the previous 12 months up to 12 weeks of unpaid leave with job protection status to care for a newborn, immediate family member (spouse or child) with a serious health issue, or deal with a personal health crisis. The US Department of Labor administers the Family and Medical Leave Act of 1993 (FMLA), and it applies to any employer of more than 50 people in a 75-mile radius. FMLA applies to any employee who worked a minimum of 1,250 hours in the previous 12 months and at least one year for the same employer. FMLA enables the employee to take up to 12 weeks of unpaid leave to care for a newborn or adopt a child. It also allows leave to care for an immediate family member (parent, spouse, or child) who suffers a serious health crisis, to care for one's own serious health issue, or certain issues with military leave. The leave can be taken all at once or intermittently. The schedule must be previously agreed upon with the employer before departure.

102. B: Americans with Disabilities Act. The Americans with Disability Act (ADA) is a federal law implemented in 1990. ADA prohibits discrimination against anyone with a disability, whether it is physical or mental impairment, or a history of the impairment. ADA is comprehensive, in that it deals with the workplace, transportation, retail establishments, restaurants, bathroom facilities, parking lots, and much more. ADA requires employers to provide reasonable accommodations to enable employees to perform their job duties in an acceptable manner. ADA also provides specific allowances for anyone who is hearing or sight impaired, or who uses assistive devices or service animals. ADA has many facets, so legal assistance is often required to ensure compliance, especially in healthcare facilities.

103. C: Behavioral interviewing. The employer's request is an example of behavioral interviewing. Behavioral interviews seek to uncover how prospective employees reacted in the past to certain types of situations, because they are likely to repeat the same behaviors in future. The benefit of a behavioral interview is as a predictor of future performance, critical thinking skills, motivation, cooperation, teamwork, and conflict resolution skills. Your interviewer expects a three-step answer from you:

1. State the situation or problem
2. Describe your action
3. Explain the result and what you learned from the situation

If you do not have any experience in dietary, then draw an example from your schooling, personal life, or unrelated jobs.

104. D: The RD meets the new employee, explains the purpose of orientation, completes the paperwork, discusses the department's purpose and objectives, introduces other employees, gives a tour of the department and overall facility, reviews Policies & Procedures, explains and demonstrates job duties, and arranges additional observation and training with a preceptor. A proper orientation reduces employee turnover and improves job performance. The orientation process prepares the new employee to perform his/her new job to an acceptable standard and to integrate smoothly with new coworkers. Orientate the new employee to the organization as a whole and then the Dietary Department. Welcome the new employee warmly. Complete the paperwork first. Explain the organizational chart; show the employee where his/her new job fits into it, and the supervisor to whom the employee will report. Review the organization's mission and departmental objectives. Take the employee on a comprehensive tour of the facility, especially restrooms, notice boards, change rooms, break rooms, and cafeteria. Point out restricted areas. Get the employee photographed for identification. Sign out necessary keys. Show the new employee the Policies & Procedures manual and give him/her a copy of necessary forms. Demonstrate his/her job duties. Allow sufficient time for observation and training, so the employee can perform job duties safely and effectively.

105. A: An opportunity for the employee to demand more salary, regardless of the details of the appraisal. Although the performance appraisal is the time when pay raises, promotions, or transfers, are awarded, its primary objective is not to obtaining more money or a more desirable position. Ideally, the PA is a way to review the employee's past performance and set his/her course for the future. Identify the employee's strengths and weaknesses. Gently point out any performance standards that have not been met. Agree on a plan that will help the employee address these weak areas. Set goals and objectives for the coming year. The PA is a good opportunity for the employee and manager to meet one-on-one, to discuss performance and other pertinent issues, such as tuition bursaries and time off for classes and teach-back.

106. B: Most production and inventory FTEs are scheduled during off-peak hours Monday to Friday, leaving a few FTE's for mealtimes and weekends. A cook-chill system streamlines the scheduling process. Many FTE's required for production and inventory can be scheduled Monday to Friday, leaving a limited number of FTE's for rethermalization and patient service. Cook-chill also helps the RD to tailor the schedule to provide more flexible shifts for employee satisfaction. Often times, the early morning and weekend production shifts are undesirable to employees. Therefore, the RD can adjust the shifts to give most full-time staff the weekends off, and schedule students and part-timers on the weekends. The overall schedule is not directly related to the tray line operation. Cook-chill allows you to schedule employees for when they are needed, with less down time. For example, employees can be scheduled for a 3-hour meal service shift. Production employees do not rush to prepare food for tray line operation, to be served immediately, which can reduce accidents.

107. D: All of the above. The three types of schedules that a food service manager is responsible for writing are the master schedule, shift schedule, and production schedule. The master schedule is written on a set rotation, such as every two weeks or every three weeks. The master schedule indicates employees' days off and vacation time. Include the weekend rotation on the master schedule; do not separate weekdays from weekends. Ensure kitchen work gets done in the most cost-effective way. For example, do not allow all cooks to take the same week off as vacation, so that you do not pay for overtime coverage unnecessarily. Base the shift schedule on the master schedule. The shift schedule lets the employees know the hours they will work. The production schedule lets the employees know their daily tasks and the period for completion.

108. D: Unions require all employees to join if the workplace is an open shop. Junior dietitians may be union members. Senior dietitians are usually management. Kitchen staff are often union members. The usual reasons for employees to join a union are dissatisfaction with management rules and policies, low compensation, and lack of job satisfaction. Membership in a union protects workers from unfair management practices or management decisions made unjustifiably. Examples of union protection are unfair dismissal cases or job demotion without a sound reason. Union negotiators can help secure higher pay and improved benefits packages in employment contracts. There are federal laws to protect an employee regarding unions:

- If the workplace is an open shop, the employee is not required to join the union
- If the workplace is an agency shop, the employee does not have to join but does pay dues, even if he/she is not a member
- If the workplace is a union shop, the employee must join the union after a certain amount of time on the job, usually three to six months

109. B: Labor budget. A Total Budget has four parts: The Operating Budget, Cash Budget, Capital Budget, and Master Budget. The Operating Budget is the quantity of sales, expenses, and revenue that is predicted for a certain period of time, usually one fiscal year, which does not necessarily begin in January and end in December. The Cash Budget is the predicted cash flow to ensure money is available when financial obligations must be met. The Capital Budget is the amount of money planned for equipment, buildings, groundskeeping, or renovations. The Master Budget puts all these pieces together to provide the organization's Financial Plan. If you are responsible for kitchen finances, ask the accountant assigned to Dietary to outline your department's financial picture when you start your new job, and again at six-month intervals.

110. A: Interpersonal, technical, conceptual. The three main skills that make an effective manager, who is likely to be promoted, are interpersonal, technical, and conceptual. Interpersonal skills help the manager relate to people and to understand different behaviors. Communication skills fall into the interpersonal category. Conceptual skills help the manager see the organization's 'big picture', rather than just what affects the kitchen. Conceptualization helps the manager evaluate how many different issues relate to each other in the end. Technical skills are specific planning and kitchen skills required for the area the manager oversees. The manager's technical skills must be well rounded, so that he/she can be seconded to work in more than one area during periods of short staffing. The RD must understand and analyze both kitchen and business processes to effectively evaluate and manage the operation.

111. B: The means to increasing productivity and efficiency is through process improvement. The classical style of management developed during the Industrial Revolution (ca. 1760-1830). It evolved from the belief that managers must find the best way to perform a certain function. Classical management theory focuses on employees completing tasks assigned to them by managers. Classical management theorists include Frederick Taylor, Frank and Lillian Gilbreth, and

Max Weber. Taylor looked at process improvement as a way to increase productivity. The Gilbreths performed time-motion studies, developed procedures, and trained employees in the more productive procedures. Weber believed all organizations needed common characteristics, such as a hierarchy of control, standard policies and procedures, and division of responsibilities, so each employee knows exactly what to do for his/her own job.

112. C: Behavioral. Maslow's Hierarchy of Needs is the basis of Behavioral Management Theory. Abraham Maslow (1908-1970) was a psychologist who believed people are:

- Never totally satisfied
- Ultimately motivated by their need to be satisfied
- Driven by their needs in order of importance

According to Maslow, the five basic needs are physiological, safety, social, esteem, and self-actualization, in that specific order. Physiological needs mean adequate food, water, and warmth. Safety means freedom from fear and a basic sense of security. Social needs include love, acceptance, belonging, and establishing deep relationships with others. Esteem means developing self-confidence and achieving a certain status or level of fame. Self-actualization means personal growth and development, which can only be met after all four previous levels of the hierarchy. Since Dietary meets the physiological needs of patients, it ranks highly and is vital to the organization.

113. D: A clinical RD dates another RD, who is the assistant manager in the food production area. The American Dietetic Association developed a voluntary Code of Ethics for RD's. The Code of Ethics outlines the values and morals that guide the profession, maintain its credibility, and protect the consumer. In the examples cited, any dietetics professional who tries to sell a product to clients for financial gain, without full disclosure, violates the Code of Ethics. Any type of substance abuse on the job, including prescription painkillers, is a violation because it could lead the RD to miscalculate sensitive ingredients, such as sugar levels for diabetics. A bipolar RD who refuses treatment and continues to practice could endanger herself or others, and thereby violates the Code of Ethics. However, two RD's with different jobs in the same organization who date are not necessarily violating the Code, unless one is in a position of authority over the other, or sexual harassment is involved.

114. A: State licensure laws define the term nutritionist and the scope varies greatly. Only candidates who pass the dietetic registration examination can legally use the title Registered Dietitian, and they must remain in good standing with the Commission on Accreditation for Dietetics Education. The use of the term registered dietitian (RD) or diet technician, registered (DTR) is tightly regulated by the Commission on Accreditation for Dietetics Education (CADE). Misuse of either title can result in legal action. RDs complete specific academic requirements and a supervised practice in the form of an internship or didactic program. The RD passes a national registration exam and is in good standing with CADE. The RD keeps current by fulfilling a continuing education requirement, required to maintain registration. By contrast, the term nutritionist varies widely by education requirements. Some nutritionists may actually have no formal training or education in nutrition. Many states enacted licensure laws to help define who is entitled to use the title nutritionist. Consumers are safest consulting an RD or DTR for credible nutrition advice.

115. C: Employees must follow their job descriptions with minimal variation from procedure. Total quality management (TQM) is a strategy to improve customer satisfaction through best practices. W. Edwards Deming created TQM. TQM was used heavily in the 1990s but has gradually evolved to quality improvement. The bottom line remains customer satisfaction.

Teamwork is integral to the success of TQM. A facilitator, usually the facility's CPHQ, moves the process forward. The facilitator empowers employees and encourages them to suggest better ways to accomplish tasks. The CPHQ, Quality Assurance Manager, Risk Manager, and Infection Control Practitioner analyze workflows closely. Explain to the staff that the goals of a TQM review are to eliminate waste and continuous improvement. The steps of TQM are: Identify the problem; determine the possible causes; develop measurable and identifiable improvements; implement a solution; measure outcomes; fine tune the improvement through feedback. Emphasize to your staff that the QA team scrutinizes flaws in the process. The QA team does not seek to lay blame on individuals.

116. B: Benchmarking. Press Ganey Associates, Inc. is a company that provides benchmarking data to food service organizations. Benchmarking compares the team's current performance against those who are widely considered to be the best. Press Ganey distributes satisfaction questionnaires to patients who received inpatient hospital care or who used outpatient services. Press Ganey performs a comparative analysis for all healthcare facilities that participate in this benchmarking process. Press Ganey owns an extensive database and validates its results. Benchmarking is a tool that food service operations can use to help improve overall patient/customer satisfaction.

117. A: Tracer process. The Joint Commission oversees a voluntary accreditation process. The mission of the Joint Commission is to ensure patient safety and a high standard for quality of care. In 2004, the Joint Commission changed the way it conducts its surveys to the tracer process. The Joint Commission selects certain patients and follows the care the patient receives throughout his or her hospital stay or outpatient clinic visits. All care, services, procedures, and tests are evaluated for quality and adherence to regulations, such as safety initiatives. The Joint Commission evaluates the relationships between various departments and disciplines for continuity and patient focus. For example, the Joint Commission looks at how Dietary, Biochemistry, and Nursing interact to provide diabetics with the correct diet and insulin.

118. B: 10.0 mg of Lipitor QD. The Joint Commission developed a Do Not Use List to reduce potential medication errors due to unclear or erroneous documentation. "10.0 mg of Lipitor QD" breaches the Do Not Use List in five ways:

- Including the decimal point in 10.0 — If the nurse misses the decimal point, an incorrect dose of 100 could be delivered.
- Unacceptable abbreviation — The nurse or pharmacist could mistake QD for QOD, so the doctor should write out "daily" for clarity.
- Obsolete abbreviation — The US prefers the unit "mL" over "cc" since the 1970s.
- Confusing abbreviation — Write out morphine sulfate because it can be confused with magnesium sulfate.
- Illegible abbreviation — Write out International Units instead of abbreviating to IU because it can be mistaken for IV (intravenous) or the number 10.

119. C: Change menu prices in the employee cafeteria all at once, rather than one at a time. To control or reduce food costs:

- Reduce theft by setting up security measures in tempting areas
- Buy seasonal items and plan meals around cheap and abundant produce
- Rotate inventory so it does not spoil, thereby decreasing discards
- Create standardized recipes and do not add extraneous ingredients to recipes
- Use portion control

- Schedule production for the greatest efficiency
- Create par levels for ingredients to avoid too much or too little of a product being prepared
- Implement price increases gradually, to prevent loyal customers from getting angry and taking their business elsewhere

120. B: Ask each worker to relate his/her version of events calmly. Restate the issue in your own words. Get additional information. Mutually agree on what the problem actually is. Brainstorm possible resolutions. Negotiate an acceptable resolution for both of them. Always conduct conflict resolution calmly and patiently. Show both parties respect. Convey that you understand the situation by rephrasing it in your own words. Use active listening skills and assertiveness. Obtain any additional information you require to clarify the situation, such as checking old schedules to identify an attendance pattern. Get both parties to agree on what the problem really is, then make them work together to find possible solutions. Negotiate to ensure everyone is satisfied with the outcome. Remember, conflict in the workplace is dangerous and should not be ignored. Kitchen tools can be weapons and there is an opportunity for poisoning. The manager's positive attitude is leadership in the right direction. If you think a threat is likely to become a reality, then you are legally liable to report the situation to the police.

121. D: Popularity of the item in the cafeteria. Generally, when a customer evaluates a meal's quality, the popularity of one item with other customers is not a primary factor. However, the customer may initially select the food item based on what other customers are ordering in his/her presence. The customer assesses the meal's quality according to: How the meal tastes; acceptability of portion size; how the food was prepared, and overall service. A food service operation cannot hide the use of low-quality food. Food specifications spell out exactly the quality that is expected, including food grade, form, pack, and price. If a miserable cashier is the last food service employee the customer sees, then it negatively influences the customer's opinion of the meal, even if the food was of good quality.

122. A: Entrance interviews. The food service manager can evaluate the food service operation by customer perception. Customers determine if they are satisfied as they are eating. Entrance interviews do not capture any real information because the customer has not yet selected food and eaten it. Exit interviews or talking to customers in the dining area are preferable ways to obtain useful information. However, personal exit interviews are difficult when the customer is ready to leave for an appointment. Use customer surveys or customer comment cards, instead. Hand the cards to customers as they leave and ask them to return the cards at a specific place, like an anonymous suggestion box. Limit the card to a few questions. All customers should answer exactly the same questions. Usually, only customers who are very happy or very upset complete a survey. Therefore, the results could be skewed.

123. C: Gender. The four factors that most influence an employee's level of job satisfaction are personality, values, overall work environment, and social influences. Personality is the top indicator. A generally happy person, who is satisfied with his/her overall life, is typically a good, productive worker. Values related to the job itself and the outcome of the work depend on the worker's culture of origin and the corporate culture. The work environment includes the physical facility, the hours of work, salary, benefits, and coworkers on the same team. Social influences include the status conferred by the job and the culture of the organization. For example, the organization that values hard-working employees and rewards them generously is more likely to recruit and retain top chefs, dietitians, and aides than an exploitative organization that expects fast turnover. Gender is not as important as the other factors.

124. B: Factor pricing. The three most common ways to determine pricing for menu items are factor pricing, prime cost, and actual cost. Factor pricing involves determining a factor that will be used as the mark-up. Typically, Accounting selects a percentage of the food cost as the mark-up. Multiply the raw food cost by the pricing factor to get the menu sales price. Do not take direct labor costs into account when factor pricing. The prime cost involves the raw food cost and the direct labor cost of producing the item. General assumptions are made to determine various factors, so the labor cost does not need to be calculated for each food item. Actual cost involves determining the cost of the item using standardized recipes, adding labor costs and any other variable costs, to determine the price point.

125. B: Authoritarian. Several leadership styles can be used to manage employees. In this case, the Clinical Nutrition Manager demonstrates an Authoritarian or Autocratic style of leadership. It is one of the least effective styles. The manager strictly enforces policies and procedures, and makes decisions independently, without input from employees. The Participative style gives rewards for good work and is more democratic. Participative style is usually a more effective style of leading. The manager invites input from employees but still has the final say in any decision making. Delegative style is also known as Laissez-Faire. The manager does not give real guidance to employees. Decisions are not made exclusively by the manager. Roles are not well defined. Motivation among employees is not very strong.

Practice Test #2

1. A critical antecedent to the NCPM is:

    a. the physician's diagnosis.

    b. evidenced-based data.

    c. a referral.

    d. the diet history.

2. The NCPM is designed for use with all EXCEPT:

    a. clients.

    b. RDs.

    c. groups.

    d. patients.

3. Which process is not typically completed by an RD?

    a. Analysis of data

    b. Identification of the problem(s)

    c. Evaluation of outcomes

    d. Performance of the nutritional screening

4. Within the NCPM, a well-written nutritional diagnostic statement is all of the following EXCEPT:

    a. related to observations by interdisciplinary team.

    b. clear and concise.

    c. accurately related to etiology.

    d. nonjudgmental.

5. Elements of the nutritional care plan implementation in the NCPM include all of the following EXCEPT:

    a. the formulation of goals.

    b. care delivery.

    c. a review with a physician for approval.

    d. documentation.

6. The vision for the combined tools of NCPM and IDNT was that they should do all of the following EXCEPT:

    a. make the RD's work my easy and efficient.

    b. enable a more accurate description of nutrition problems.

    c. describe the results of nutritional interventions.

    d. facilitate medical documentation.

7. A primary use of the IDNT is:

    a. to get other health care providers involved in nutritional care.

    b. to document nutritional care in the medical record.

    c. to get reimbursement for nutritional care.

    d. to develop a logic model for nutritional care.

8. In the INDT, the development of diagnostic language includes all the following domains EXCEPT:
   a. food and/or nutritional intake.
   b. clinical.
   c. medical.
   d. behavioral/environmental.

9. The purpose of NCP is to:
   a. optimize nutrition-related outcomes.
   b. increase communication with an interdisciplinary team.
   c. establish the importance of the RD in patient care.
   d. demonstrate the need for nutrition management.

10. When used with computerized systems, standardized terminologies such as IDNT support accurate:
   a. diagnosis.
   b. communication.
   c. data entry and analysis.
   d. decision making.

11. External factors affecting the IDNT Logic Model include:
   a. medical and nursing language.
   b. current health care media.
   c. institution or practice.
   d. health care policy, legislation, and regulation.

12. Before a nutritional diagnosis can be accepted for general use, it must undergo:
   a. reliability testing.
   b. content validation.
   c. approval from the American Medical Association.
   d. interdisciplinary validation.

13. All of the following are categories of a nutritional assessment EXCEPT:
   a. clinical data.
   b. physical findings.
   c. etiology.
   d. nutrition history.

14. Elements of critical thinking in the nutrition assessment include:
   a. making interdisciplinary plans.
   b. prioritizing.
   c. selecting appropriate indicators.
   d. validating data.

15. The purpose of the nutrition diagnosis in the NCP is to:
   a. identify a specific nutrition problem.
   b. validate the referring diagnosis.
   c. validate the nutritional assessment.
   d. formulate a care plan.

16. What is the best phrase to link the etiology to the diagnosis?

   a. "Caused by…"
   b. "Related to…"
   c. "Following…"
   d. "Data show…"

17. A nutrition intervention should most importantly:

   a. educate patients about their nutritional needs.
   b. consider the patient's socioeconomic and cultural background.
   c. resolve or improve the patient's nutritional problem.
   d. validate the nutritional diagnosis.

18. In the NCP, the determination of the nutritional intervention is primarily guided by the:

   a. prioritizing nutrition diagnosis.
   b. patient's education level.
   c. environmental conditions.
   d. nutrition diagnosis and etiology.

19. All of the following are factors affecting nutritional requirements EXCEPT:

   a. infection and fever.
   b. disease.
   c. socioeconomics.
   d. psychological stress.

20. In the nutrition monitoring and evaluation phase of the NCP, all of the following are elements EXCEPT:

   a. nutrition-related history outcomes.
   b. biochemical data.
   c. anthropometrics.
   d. signs and symptoms.

21. In metabolic syndrome, all the risk factors are primarily related to:

   a. hypertension.
   b. type 2 diabetes.
   c. obesity.
   d. cardiovascular disease.

22. Trans fatty acids should be _____ of total caloric intake.

   a. <15%
   b. <10%
   c. <5%
   d. <1%

23. In the NCP, PES stands for:

   a. Patient, Estimated, Status.
   b. Problem, Etiology, Symptoms.
   c. Principal, Etiology, Signs.
   d. Problem, Evaluation, Statement.

24. In the monitoring and evaluation step of the NCP, indication that new needs have arisen prompts:

    a. restatement of the diagnosis, including the new problem.
    b. expansion of the evaluation to include the new problem.
    c. incorporation of the new problem into the care plan.
    d. restarting the NCP.

25. Examples of a nutrition diagnosis within the NCP using the IDNT include all of the following EXCEPT:

    a. inadequate oral food/beverage intake.
    b. disordered eating pattern.
    c. hypermetabolism.
    d. altered GI function.

26. In the A-D-I-M-E chart content, M stands for:

    a. measurement.
    b. management.
    c. monitoring.
    d. medication.

27. In the nutrition assessment, the RD should be aware that obesity is associated with certain markers for coronary heart disease, including all the following EXCEPT:

    a. elevated sodium and potassium.
    b. low grade inflammatory state.
    c. C-reactive protein.
    d. cytokines.

28. Nutritional screening identifies those at nutritional risk. The most import factors affecting nutritional risk include all the following EXCEPT:

    a. food intake patterns.
    b. psychosocial factors.
    c. social factors, such as family size.
    d. associated diseases and disorders.

29. Essential elements of the nutrition assessment includes:

    a. determining the intervention.
    b. identifying and appropriate MNT.
    c. determining BMI.
    d. establishing nutritional goals.

30. Nutritional goals are primarily part of the:

    a. nutrition screening.
    b. nutrition intervention.
    c. nutrition diagnosis.
    d. nutrition outcome.

31. Rationales for choosing enteral nutrition support include all the following EXCEPT:
    a. the need to preserve gastrointestinal immunity.
    b. the need to preserve pulmonary mucosal immunity.
    c. inadequate oral intake to maintain optimal nutritional status.
    d. patient with at least five to six feet of functioning small bowel.

32. Standard enteral formulas contain what percent of lipid?
    a. 10-20%
    b. 20-30%
    c. 30-40%
    d. 40-50%

33. Nonessential amino acids for standard parenteral nutrition are supplied by:
    a. glutamine and arginine.
    b. alanine and glycine.
    c. glutamate and cysteine.
    d. taurine and homocysteine.

34. At a BMI of 27-35, the NIH suggests a weight loss of:
    a. 0.5-1.0 lb/wk.
    b. 1.0-2.0 lb/wk.
    c. 2.5-3.0 lb/wk.
    d. 3.5-4.0 lb/wk.

35. Morbid obesity is described as a BMI of:
    a. 25 or more.
    b. 30 or more.
    c. 35 or more.
    d. 40 or more.

36. The goal of treatment for an overweight child is:
    a. weight loss of 1 lb per month.
    b. weight loss of 2 lb per month.
    c. weight maintenance.
    d. weight loss of 0.5 lb per month.

37. Which of the following is characteristic of only type 1 diabetes mellitus?
    a. Autoantibodies
    b. Insulin resistance
    c. Hypoglycemia
    d. Insulin requiring

38. Type 2 diabetes may account for what percent of all diabetes mellitus?
    a. 50-60%
    b. 60-75%
    c. 75-90%
    d. 90-95%

39. Which nutrition diagnosis is not related to diabetes mellitus?

a. Excessive energy intake
b. Intake of unsafe foods
c. Altered GI function
d. Disordered eating pattern

40. The best test to determine hypoglycemia is:

a. GTT.
b. A1c.
c. SMBG.
d. Fasting blood glucose.

41. A 67-year-old man weighs 190 pounds and is 5 feet 9 inches tall. According to his BMI, he is:

a. underweight.
b. healthy.
c. overweight.
d. obese.

42. Chronic pancreatitis treatment requires supplements of all of the following EXCEPT:

a. vitamin C.
b. pancreatic enzymes.
c. fat-soluble vitamins.
d. vitamin B_{12}.

43. The chief nutritional finding in cirrhosis of the liver is:

a. hypoglycemia.
b. ascites.
c. hyperglycemia.
d. malnutrition.

44. The glycemic index uses which of the following as a standard for comparison?

a. Sucrose
b. Fructose
c. White bread
d. Potato

45. MNT for heart failure includes all of the following EXCEPT:

a. increased use of whole grains, fruits, and vegetables.
b. sodium restriction.
c. fluid restriction.
d. vitamin B_{12} supplementation.

46. At the onset of acute renal failure, the nutritional treatment of choice is often:

a. fluid, protein, and sodium restriction.
b. TPN.
c. fluid and sodium restriction.
d. enteral feeding modified in protein and electrolytes.

47. Nutritional goals of end-stage renal disease include all the following EXCEPT:

a. preventing uremia with significant protein restriction.
b. preventing nutritional deficiencies.
c. controlling edema and serum electrolytes.
d. preventing renal osteodystrophy.

48. Metabolic/medical complications of HIV include all the following EXCEPT:

a. diabetes mellitus.
b. hyperlipidemia.
c. osteoporosis.
d. urticaria.

49. Addition of which substance is the most commonly recommended in MNT of many psychiatric disorders?

a. Vitamin D
b. Omega-3 fatty acids
c. Vitamin B_6
d. Polyunsaturated oils

50. What measurement of obesity indicates a risk for metabolic syndrome, diabetes, and heart disease?

a. RMS
b. Skinfold thickness
c. Waist circumference
d. BMI

51. Models for behavior change include all of the following EXCEPT:

a. psychosocial behavior analysis.
b. transtheoretical model of change.
c. motivational interviewing.
d. cognitive behavioral therapy.

52. Factors that influence one's willingness to make nutritional changes include all the following EXCEPT:

a. readiness.
b. nutritionist's style.
c. education level.
d. ambivalence.

53. What model or approach for behavioral change relates thinking to behavior?

a. Cognitive behavioral therapy
b. Transtheoretical model
c. Motivational interviewing
d. Reflective listening

54. Which of the following does not describe a characteristic of the adult learner?

   a. Self-directed
   b. Goal-oriented
   c. Sequential
   d. Relevancy-oriented

55. In order to help patients develop motivation, the dietitian must do all the following EXCEPT:

   a. enhance reasons for learning.
   b. decrease barriers to learning.
   c. present the material so that it is relevant to the patients' lives.
   d. remind patients that for health reasons they must make this dietary change.

56. A good teaching activity for a newly diabetic patient would be which of the following?

   a. Making a list of all the bad things he eats
   b. Constructing a meal from his diabetic meal plan
   c. Memorizing a list of foods high on the glycemic index
   d. Developing an entirely new eating schedule to match his diagnosis

57. What are the key elements in motivational interviewing?

   a. Persuasion and support
   b. Motivation and feedback
   c. Cultural and social understanding
   d. Inspiration and teaching skill

58. All of the following are designated areas for research by Academy of Nutrition and Dietetics EXCEPT:

   a. public health.
   b. clinical nutrition research.
   c. suitable IT development.
   d. implementation science.

59. A priority area of nutrition-related discovery is:

   a. nutrition problems in gene-specific chemotherapy.
   b. interventions to prevent and treat obesity and other chronic diseases.
   c. updates on TPN.
   d. the role of the dietitian in an interdisciplinary team.

60. To be an effective multicultural communicator, the dietitian must be aware of all of the following EXCEPT:

   a. vocabulary.
   b. eye contact.
   c. eating habits.
   d. intelligence.

61. **Nutritional goals should be all of the following EXCEPT:**
    a. achievable.
    b. focused on the short term.
    c. set by the dietitian according to diagnosis.
    d. the basis of a plan.

62. **Which is the most important counseling session?**
    a. The first session, in which the dietitian establishes rapport
    b. The second session, in which the dietitian presents vital information
    c. The third session, in which the patient completes learning tasks
    d. The fourth and last session, in which the dietitian summarizes the information, takes questions, and reestablishes goals

63. **The following are all enzymes secreted in the small intestine EXCEPT:**
    a. sucrase.
    b. nucleotidases.
    c. amylase.
    d. enterokinase.

64. **What is the area of the absorptive surface of the small intestine?**
    a. 3 mi²
    b. 10 m²
    c. 200-300 m²
    d. 500-600 ft

65. **All the following factors affect resting energy expenditure EXCEPT:**
    a. body composition.
    b. activity level.
    c. sex.
    d. hormone status.

66. **Which of the following is not a monosaccharide?**
    a. Sucrose
    b. Glucose
    c. Dextrose
    d. Galactose

67. **Major regulators of blood glucose after a meal include all of the following EXCEPT:**
    a. the amount of digestible carbohydrate.
    b. uptake and absorption by the liver.
    c. insulin secretion and tissue sensitivity to it.
    d. the level on the glycemic index.

68. **Approximately how much of portal glucose is taken up by the liver?**
    a. 20%
    b. 30%
    c. 50%
    d. 65%

69. **Which statement about omega-3 fatty acids is TRUE?**
    a. They are synthesized by seaweed.
    b. They influence neurotransmission.
    c. They maintain the integrity of the GI tract.
    d. They are short-chain fatty acids.

70. **The absorption of vitamin E is dependent on all the following EXCEPT:**
    a. the presence of dietary fat.
    b. an adequate biliary function.
    c. a normally functioning pancreas.
    d. the presence of free radicals.

71. **What nutrient increases the need for thiamin?**
    a. alcohol
    b. whole grains
    c. yeast
    d. carbohydrate

72. **Inadequate intake of vitamin B_{12} leads to a deficiency in which of the following?**
    a. Iron
    b. Niacin
    c. Folate
    d. Vitamin B_6

73. **Iron absorption is enhanced by which of the following?**
    a. Ascorbic acid
    b. Protein
    c. Vitamin B_{12}
    d. Oxalates

74. **Factors positively affecting the absorption of calcium include all the following EXCEPT:**
    a. estrogen levels.
    b. vitamin D.
    c. high levels of exercise.
    d. low fiber diets.

75. **What are the protein requirements of an infant during the first six months of life?**
    a. 8 g/day
    b. 9 g/day
    c. 11 g/day
    d. 12 g/day

Use the following restaurant meal for questions 76 and 77:

- 2 roasted chicken legs
- 1 cup fettuccine alfredo
- 1 cup broccoli with 1 tsp butter
- Salad greens with 2 tbsp of Italian dressing
- 2 dinner rolls with 2 tsp butter
- 12 oz white wine
- Coffee with 2 tbsp of half & half
- ½ cup chocolate ice cream

76. Approximately how many calories are in this meal?
   a. 800-1000
   b. 1100-1300
   c. 1400-1600
   d. 1700-1900

77. Approximately how many grams of fat are in this meal?
   a. 30-50
   b. 51-85
   c. 86-110
   d. 111-130

78. What is the acronym for a storage and stock rotation principle?
   a. LILO
   b. FIFO
   c. APPM
   d. SSRP

79. Which of the following is a variable cost?
   a. Labor
   b. Equipment
   c. Insurance
   d. Utilities

80. An ideal storage location will have all of the following effects EXCEPT:
   a. reducing labor requirements.
   b. speeding the storing and issuing of food.
   c. minimizing security risks.
   d. decreasing transit time between the preparation and serving areas.

81. Which items should be stored near the entrance of the storeroom?
   a. Freshest items
   b. First items delivered
   c. Frequently used items
   d. Perishable items

82. All the following will help prevent bacterial growth in food EXCEPT:

    a. keeping foods dry.

    b. keeping cold food at 40 °F or less.

    c. keeping hot foods at 140°F or over.

    d. not leaving food out for more than 30 minutes.

83. All the following are purposes of labor cost control EXCEPT:

    a. maximizing efficiency.

    b. preventing layoffs.

    c. using employees' services effectively.

    d. maintaining sufficient staff without down time.

84. A four-part labor cost control process would consist of all the following EXCEPT:

    a. establishing standards and standard procedures.

    b. training all staff to be aware of standards and to follow standard procedures.

    c. having every employee read the policy and procedures manual thoroughly.

    d. monitoring staff performance.

85. Factors contributing to labor costs include all following EXCEPT:

    a. age of employees.

    b. equipment.

    c. layout.

    d. menu.

86. Union contracts affect labor costs in all the following ways EXCEPT:

    a. higher wages.

    b. insurance.

    c. vacation pay.

    d. child care.

87. Which of the following is TRUE about an organizational plan?

    a. It describes each position.

    b. It requires a thorough understanding of costs.

    c. It shows reporting relationships.

    d. It shows the pathways of each operation.

88. In order to write a job description, the manager must be aware of all the following EXCEPT:

    a. job objectives.

    b. performance standards.

    c. required tasks.

    d. suggested age for the job.

89. Establishing standards and standard procedures primarily involves all of the following EXCEPT:

    a. organizing the enterprise.

    b. being aware of cost concerns.

    c. developing job descriptions.

    d. scheduling employees.

90. When would long-time employees need training?
   a. When they have been away from work on an extended sick leave
   b. When new employees have been hired
   c. When work standards or standard procedures have been changed
   d. Yearly

91. The Systems Approach states that all systems have four basic characteristics. Which of the following is not one of those characteristics?
   a. All systems have a general purpose.
   b. All systems operate within an environment.
   c. All systems have subsystems.
   d. Outside factors are an important consideration.

92. All of the following are functions of food service managers EXCEPT:
   a. monitoring staff performance.
   b. selecting and training staff.
   c. orienting staff to the interaction of union policies and department practices.
   d. preparing financial reports.

93. What are three types of food service systems?
   a. Cook chill, cook freeze, rethermalization
   b. Conventional, commissary, assembly/serve
   c. Ready-prepared, conventional, rethermalization
   d. Commissary, satellite, decentralized production

94. FAT-TOM refers to:
   a. hazardous foods.
   b. tomato selection.
   c. fast cooking method.
   d. frequent hand washing.

95. Which of the following does not cause food-borne intoxication?
   a. *Staphylococcus aureus*
   b. *Listeria monocytogenes*
   c. *Clostridium botulinum*
   d. *Clostridium perfringens*

96. Which microorganism accounts for the most cases of GI upset?
   a. *Salmonella*
   b. *Escherichia coli*
   c. *Clostridium perfringens*
   d. *Campylobacter jejuni*

97. The role of the food service manager in food safety includes knowledge of all the following EXCEPT:
   a. symptoms associated with food-borne illness.
   b. federal, state, and local guidelines and regulations.
   c. interaction of food service employees.
   d. proper care of equipment and facilities.

98. A common food service safety education program is:

- a. OSHA.
- b. HACCP.
- c. SFS.
- d. CLEAN.

99. Barriers to a food safety program include all the following EXCEPT:

- a. federal and state regulations.
- b. lack of time and personnel.
- c. high turnover of personnel.
- d. burden of required documentation.

100. To sanitize items in a conveyor dual temperature washing machine, the water temperature should be:

- a. 150 °F.
- b. 165 °F.
- c. 175 °F.
- d. 180 °F.

101. All of the following are categories of factors affecting menu planning EXCEPT:

- a. organizational.
- b. personnel.
- c. customer.
- d. operational.

102. Which of the following is not a component of the DRI?

- a. EAR
- b. RDA
- c. WHO
- d. UL

103. All of the following describe the customer and his food needs EXCEPT:

- a. psychosocial.
- b. demographic.
- c. sociocultural.
- d. nutritional.

104. Which of the following is a food group described in the Dietary Guidelines for Americans?

- a. Proteins
- b. Vitamins
- c. Fats
- d. Minerals

105. Which kind of menu is most often used in major medical centers?

- a. Cycle
- b. Static
- c. Single use
- d. Du jour

106. In menu planning, the characteristics and combinations of foods should be considered. These include all of the following EXCEPT:

a. presentation.
b. color.
c. nutrition.
d. texture.

107. Step by step in menu planning includes all of the following EXCEPT:

a. entrées.
b. beverages.
c. vegetables.
d. sandwiches.

108. What is an extended menu?

a. One with extra items
b. One that lasts for more than one season
c. One that includes three meals and three snacks
d. One that includes modified diets

109. Elements to be considered in the printed menu include all the following EXCEPT:

a. design and format.
b. type of food served.
c. wording.
d. truth in menu legislation.

110. Theory X and Theory Y hold that managers' attitudes are of two distinct types. They are:

a. Balanced and unbalanced.
b. Optimistic and pessimistic.
c. Structured and unstructured.
d. Linear and circular.

111. What psychologist developed a hierarchy of human needs?

a. Hawthorne
b. Maslow
c. McGregor
d. Taylor

112. All the following are characteristics of good leaders EXCEPT:

a. having a strong sense of belonging to their organization.
b. questioning established procedures and creating new ones.
c. risk taking.
d. relating to people in an intuitive and empathic way.

113. A study done at Ohio State identified the characteristics employees look for in a food leader. They prefer leaders who are all of the following EXCEPT:

a. honest.
b. forward-looking.
c. in possession of a strong survival instinct.
d. competent.

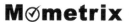

114. According to French and Raven, the specific types of power that people acquire include all the follow EXCEPT:

    a. coercive power.
    b. people power.
    c. reward power.
    d. expert power.

115. Oral communication is best used in which of the following situations?

    a. When quick action is required
    b. When employees are to be held strictly accountable
    c. When employees are inexperienced
    d. When something is being quoted

116. A leader with high ethical standards inspires all the following EXCEPT:

    a. trust.
    b. loyalty.
    c. effective leader-follower relationships.
    d. organizational respect.

117. The most important resource in any enterprise is:

    a. a well-educated and experienced manager.
    b. a strong financial base.
    c. the human factor.
    d. inspiring leadership.

118. Major marketing strategies are based on the 4 Ps. They include all of the following EXCEPT:

    a. product.
    b. persuasion.
    c. price.
    d. promotion.

119. Which of the following must be identified in order to define competition?

    a. Target market
    b. Goals
    c. Mission
    d. Objectives

120. All the following are the primary keys to successful product marketing EXCEPT:

    a. characteristics of product.
    b. product developer's image.
    c. timing in the marketplace.
    d. competitive positioning of the product.

121. All of the following scenarios show good ethical practice EXCEPT:

a. A dietitian is asked to be a consultant and spokesperson for a new artificial sweetener. She reads all the available research literature in peer-reviewed journals and decides that the product is safe and has some advantages over other artificial sweeteners.

b. A dietitian is asked to do a television interview. It is on the "Twinkie"—sugar causing adverse behavior—defense for a court case. The TV news producer wants an explanation of how sugar could cause this adverse behavior. The dietitian consults with several physicians and determines that sugar does not cause adverse behavior, so he refuses the interview.

c. A dietitian is a spokesperson for an energy bar product. The marketing department wants him to support their statement that a particular nutrient is more important than others. Although this is an exaggeration, he decides that this is a minor issue, and since the product is basically of good nutritional value, he agrees to support the marketing plan.

d. A dietitian in private practice is approached by a company that makes a diet shake that she has investigated and often recommends to patients. They offer her samples of a new product, which she evaluates and thinks is very good for dieters. The company asks her to speak at a meeting on weight loss where she does not have to endorse the product. She agrees.

122. Common pricing strategies include all the following EXCEPT:

a. skimming.
b. trading down.
c. underbidding.
d. customer specific.

123. Which of the following pieces of legislation did not deal with the acquisition of human resources?

a. Civil Rights Act of 1964
b. Occupational Safety and Health Act of 1970
c. Age Discrimination in Employment Act of 1967
d. Americans with Disabilities Act of 1990

124. All of the following are elements of the QWL approach EXCEPT:

a. work design.
b. safety and health.
c. human resources.
d. equipment design.

125. All the following are part of a Performance Improvement Plan EXCEPT:

a. updating organizational chart.
b. selecting a job to be improved.
c. breaking down the job in detail.
d. challenging every detail.

Answer Key and Explanations

1. C: A referral. The Nutrition Care Process Model (NCPM) is an approach to solving patient problems relating to nutrition. Referral occurs when a healthcare provider calls upon another practitioner to see his or her patient and to provide care beyond the scope of that provider's own practice. The term referral may also be used to describe the actual document that authorizes a visit to another health care professional and is necessary for billing purposes.

2. B: RDs. The Nutrition Care Process Model (NCPM) is designed for use with those to whom a dietitian provides nutritional care and guidance through referral. These include patients in a primary or tertiary health care setting, such as a clinic, office, or hospital and in the community. It designed for use with all ages and conditions of health or disease. The NCPM was put together after a literature review and was meant to replace previous nutritional care tools.

3. D: Performance of then nutritional screening. The nutritional screening is generally performed by another health care professional, such as a physician or a nurse, as part of the intake assessment. It occurs prior to the referral and designates patients at nutritional risk. Screening is defined as "a test or standardized examination procedure to identify patients requiring special intervention."

4. A: Related to observations by interdisciplinary team. The nutritional diagnosis is the second step in the NCPM. It follows the nutrition assessment and contains solely the observations and assessment of the RD. The nutritional diagnosis must be succinct and use the International Nutrition and Dietetics Terminology (INDT), a standard vocabulary for nutrition documentation. In this way, it is unambiguous and easily read and understood by other health care providers. The nutritional diagnosis must be correctly connected to etiology and based on the signs and symptoms of the assessment so that it follows as a logical conclusion. It must also be objective, based on data and observations in the assessment, without any personal judgment.

5. C: A review with a physician for approval. The NCPM is solely the domain of the RD and does not require physician approval. The role of the physician in the NCPM is to provide a nutritional screening and referral for nutritional intervention. The physician also collaborates with other health care professionals to provide smooth implementation of the NCP. Otherwise, implementation of the NCP involves formulation of achievable patient goals, a realistic plan for care delivery, good communication, follow-up to ensure that the plan is implemented, and modification as necessary.

6. A: Make the RD's work easier and more efficient. The International Nutrition and Dietetics Terminology (INDT) is a standard vocabulary designed to put into words each step of the NCPM and each step's data or observations. The idea for using these tools together is to aid in communication concerning nutritional care, and also to allow researchers to better document nutrition problems, care plans, and outcomes. These tools will also enhance electronic medical recordkeeping and provide information for policies, procedures, legislation, and reimbursement.

7. B: To document nutrition care in the medical record. The primary purpose of the IDNT is to document nutritional care in the patient's medical record that is clear and streamlined, minimizing confusion and standardizing the language used. According to the American Health Information Management Association, a medical record becomes a legal record of health care services received and their rationale, an avenue of communication among health care providers, and supporting documentation for reimbursement of services provided. The INDT was developed for RDs to

69

describe their nutrition-related findings and decisions within the NCPM. The use of a standardized language with a care plan will contribute to the visibility of the RD as a unique and competent provider of nutritional care and give more ready access to this information in an electronic medical record.

8. C: Medical. Diagnosis is the second of the four steps in the NCPM, which is a problem-solving model for nutritional care. The International Nutrition and Dietetics Terminology (INDT) is a standard vocabulary designed to put into words each critical step of the NCPM and each step's data or observations. The nutritional diagnosis follows the nutritional assessment and uses its findings. The food and nutrition professional is responsible for identification and labeling of an existing problem that is to be treated. According to the INDT, there are three language domains in the diagnosis section. They are food and nutrition intake, clinical, and behavioral/environmental.

9. A: Optimize nutrition-related outcomes. The Nutrition Care Process (NCP) is a problem-solving process intended for nutritional practice that was developed within the Nutrition Care Process Model (NCPM). The NCP gives the RD the ability to tailor nutritional care to specific patients, using best evidence and considering their needs and value systems. The NCP consists of four activities. The first area is assessment of nutritional status by analysis of data and physical observations to recognize nutritional problems. Following the assessment and using its data is the nutritional diagnosis. The third step is planning and prioritizing nutritional intervention to meet the patient's needs. Last is the evaluation of outcomes, determining if additional nutrition care is needed.

10. C: Data entry and analysis. The International Nutrition and Dietetics Terminology (INDT) is a standardized word set designed for use in the nutrition care process, a problem-solving method. INDT is intended for use in the electronic patient record to facilitate data entry and processing. A standardized word set, such as INDT, allows for correct data entry and analysis. When the IDNT is integrated into electronic medical records routinely and used properly, clinicians can find and retrieve specific terms and be certain that the nutrition-related term is constant in meaning, regardless of time or place.

11. D: Health care policy, legislation, and regulation. The goal of a standard nutrition language is to allow data to enhance the practice of nutrition, education, research, and policy. External factors, in addition to health care policy, regulation, and practice, affect this standard nutrition language. Subjects included are health care personnel, health insurance or Medicaid/Medicare access, regulation, and the state of the economy in the US and in the communities, medical centers, and universities. Standard nutrition language may be altered by the food supply and delivery systems and/or the effects of various subcultures.

12. B: Content validation. Nutritional diagnosis is the second of the four steps in the problem-solving process of the Nutrition Care Process Model (NCPM). The nutritional diagnosis uses the International Nutrition and Dietetics Terminology (INDT), which is a standardized word set specific to NCPM. Once diagnosis is made and found to be important, one must to establish whether it relates to real-world dietetics. Before using a term describing nutrition diagnosis, its derivation and related criteria must be seen as relevant to a nutritional state that occurs in the scope of practice. Content validation ensures that the diagnostic terms and their related vocabulary actually exist in dietetic practice and that RDs have the experience and ability to utilize them.

13. C: Etiology. Nutrition assessment is the first step of the nutrition care process (NCP), which is a nutrition problem- solving system. Nutrition assessment data are organized into five categories. The first is food/nutrition-related history, including food, supplement and medicine intake, knowledge and beliefs, food supply, and activity level. The next area is biochemical data, medical tests, and procedures. The third area is anthropometric measurements and client history, including personal history, medical health/family history, alternative medicine use, and social history.

14. D: Validating data. The purpose of the nutrition assessment is to obtain, verify, interpret, and record data needed to identify nutrition-related problems, their causes, and significance. Critical thinking steps for the nutrition assessment include

- Deciding what data to collect
- Choosing appropriate assessment tools and procedures and using them correctly
- Deciding what data is relevant
- Distinguishing important from unimportant data
- Validating the data collected and analyzed

15. A: Identify a specific nutrition problem. The purpose of the nutrition diagnosis is to identify and describe a specific nutrition condition that the RD can address and correct or ameliorate through nutrition treatment/ intervention. The nutrition diagnosis is determined by utilizing the information gained in the nutritional assessment. It is different from a medical diagnosis (for example, gallbladder disease) in that rather than relating to a medical condition, it relates to a dietary pattern (such as high fat intake). The nutrition diagnosis is made using the standard terminology as defined by International Nutrition and Dietetics Terminology (IDNT).

16. B: "Related to". The diagnosis labels a specific nutritional condition. Etiology refers to the factors that cause disease and how the patient acquired that disease. In the NCP, the nutritional diagnosis is linked to a medical cause and contributing factors. According to the Nutritional Care Plan model (NCPM) and the International Nutrition and Dietetics Terminology (IDNT), the best way to link the etiology to the nutritional diagnosis is by using the phrase "related to."

17. C: Resolve or improve the patient's nutritional problem. Nutrition intervention is the third step in the Nutrition Care Process (NCP), which is a nutrition problem- solving system. The purpose of nutrition Intervention is to correct or ameliorate the identified nutrition problem by planning and implementing appropriate nutrition interventions tailored to the patient's specific needs. Nutrition intervention strategies are purposely selected to change nutritional intake, nutrition-related knowledge or behavior, environmental conditions, or access to supportive care and services. Nutrition intervention establishes goals by which to monitor and measure progress. These goals may be changed or modified, depending on outcome

18. D: Nutrition diagnosis and etiology. In the Nutrition Care Process (NCP), which is a nutrition problem solving system, diagnosis establishes the nutritional problem, and etiology includes the factors that cause the problem. The two terms represent the problem and the source of the problem, so they are the primary drivers in determining the nutrition intervention most suitable to the patient. The nutritional diagnosis and etiology are key in the process of developing and delivering nutrition education. They determine the type of education, nutrient (i.e., carbohydrate, fat, or sodium) to be modified. Also, the approach to the educational process is driven by these factors. Did the patient become obese and develop diabetes, or is a sodium-modified food intake advised as a precaution in the development of heart disease?

19. C: Socioeconomics. Nutritional requirements are affected by many physiological and psychological factors. These factors differ from factors affecting food intake. While food intake depends on a wide number of issues, including environmental, psychosocial, and physiological, nutritional requirements reflect the physiologic and psychological state of the individual's body.

Infection and fever may cause an anabolic state, increasing metabolism and nutritional needs. Diseases of the GI tract may cause limited absorption of nutrients, increasing requirements for nutrients. GI disorders may also cause blockage or another altered state in the stomach or intestines, necessitating a change of food consistency. Diabetes causes altered glucose metabolism, demanding a modified meal plan timed to complement medication, with limitations on carbohydrate in the diet as well as on overall calories. Psychological stress may cause an inability to consume food, leading to a malnourished state.

20. D: Signs and symptoms. Nutrition monitoring and evaluation is the fourth and final step in the Nutrition Care Process (NCP), which is a problem-solving system for nutritional care. The purpose of nutrition evaluation and monitoring is to determine the amount of progress made by the patient/client and whether goals/expected outcomes are being met. Nutrition monitoring and evaluation identifies patient/client outcomes relevant to the nutrition diagnosis, intervention, plans, and goals. The four elements of the nutrition monitoring and evaluation are food/nutrition-related history outcomes, pertinent biochemical data and test results, anthropometric measurement, and nutrition-focused physical finding outcomes.

21. C: Obesity. Metabolic syndrome is increasingly common and is even seen in children. It is a name for a group of risk factors that occur together and increase the risk for the development of coronary artery disease, stroke, and type 2 diabetes. This group of risk factors includes obesity, insulin resistance, hypertriglyceridemia, low HDL cholesterol, and hypertension. All the other factors are related to obesity, with abdominal obesity being the most outstanding symptom. Diagnosis is made when three or more of the above factors are present.

22. B: < 10%. Of all the dietary fats, trans fatty acids have the most significant negative impact on serum lipids. Trans fatty acids occur when polyunsaturated fats are partially hydrogenated, as in the hardening of oil into margarine. The hydrogenation of vegetable oils produces elaidic acid, the most common trans fatty acid. Other sources include hydrogenated/partially hydrogenated vegetable oils that are used to make shortening and commercially prepared baked goods, snack foods, and fried foods. The most common naturally occurring trans fatty acid is trans-vaccenic acid found in animals (e.g., beef, and lamb) and dairy products. The RDA suggests that less than 10% of caloric intake come from trans fatty acids.

23. B: Problem, etiology, symptoms. The PES statement refers to problem, etiology, and symptoms. It is a way to organize the information relating to the nutritional diagnosis. Problem refers to the nutritional diagnosis and etiology and symptoms are the history/derivation and presentation of the nutritional diagnosis respectively. It is part of second step in the Nutrition Care Process (NCP), which is a problem-solving system for nutritional care. It utilizes the Nutrition and Dietetics Terminology (INDT), a nutrition specific standard language.

24. D: Restart the NCP. Monitoring and evaluation determine whether the nutritional goals are being met and identify outcomes relevant to the nutrition diagnosis and intervention. It is possible that the monitoring and evaluation phase may reveal nutritional problems not previously seen. At this point it is necessary to start the NCP over again. A new assessment is needed to verify, analyze, and translate the data relevant to new the nutritional problem, its causes, and importance. A second nutritional diagnosis may be determined if the new problem is either related or unrelated to the first nutrition diagnosis. After establishing a new nutrition diagnosis, the dietitian continues with a new NCP.

25. C: Hypermetabolism. Hypermetabolism was one of the original diagnoses proposed by the Academy of American Dietetics. In a validation study published in 2008, Enrione suggested that nutrition terms for diagnoses should be submitted for validation. It needs to be established that identified terminology/concepts exist in real-world dietetics and can be treated by a dietitian. The term hypermetabolism was dropped from the list because it was decided that dietitians were unable to treat this diagnosis.

26. C: Monitoring. The A-D-I-M-E chart allows the dietitian to organize the nutrition information of Nutrition Care Process (NCP), a problem-solving system for nutritional care, in a consistent way in the patient's medical record. A stands for assessment, D stands for diagnosis, I for intervention, and M/E for monitoring and evaluation. Monitoring and evaluation comprise the fourth step in the NCP. It is this step that decides whether the nutritional goals are satisfied and identifies outcomes relating to the nutritional diagnosis. There are four types of outcomes that are reported by the RD: food/nutrition history and knowledge, biochemical data, tests and procedures, and anthropometric measurements, such as height, weight, and BMI, along with nutrition-related physical findings, including appearance, muscle and fat wasting, swallow function, appetite, and affect.

27. A: Elevated sodium and potassium. Overnutrition presents major nutritional problems leading to obesity, diabetes, atherosclerotic disease, and metabolic syndrome. The injured obese patient may present some difficulties that put him or her at a unique risk, because current nutrition assessment tools screen only for undernourishment, not over-nourishment. Thus, the injured obese patient is recorded as being at no or minimal nutritional risk and is less likely to be screened over time, resulting in the potential for increased morbidity. The RD should be aware that obesity is associated with a low-grade inflammatory state and the presence of inflammatory markers such as C-reactive protein and proinflammatory cytokines. This inflammatory state results in comorbidities such as heart disease. More appropriate tools are needed to accurately assess this population.

28. C: Social factors, such as family size. Screening for nutritional risk takes place before for the Nutrition Care Process (NCP), a problem-solving system for nutritional care. It is usually carried out by a physician or health care professional other than the RD. Nutrition screening quickly identifies those who are malnourished or otherwise at nutritional risk and determines whether a more complete nutritional assessment is needed. The most important factors affecting nutritional risk include

- Food intake patterns
- Psychosocial factors
- Physical conditions associated diseases and disorders
- Biochemical abnormalities
- Medication regimens

Psychosocial factors would include social factors, such as family composition.

29. C: Determining BMI. The nutrition assessment is the first step in the nutritional a care plan (NCP), a problem-solving system for nutritional care. It is a comprehensive evaluation carried out by the RD for defining nutritional status using medical, social, nutritional, and medication histories; anthropometric measurements; and lab data. The body mass index or BMI is one of the anthropometric measurements and a validated measure of nutrition status. It is used to describe the degree of adiposity. The metric formula for BMI is $(kg)/ht(m)^2$. The English formula is $lb/(ht[in])^2 \times 703$.

30. B: Nutrition intervention. Once nutritional diagnosis is established, intervention can begin. The nutritional goals are an essential element in the intervention step of the NCP. They determine what nutritional objectives should be met to treat the diagnosis and what educational format and counseling process should be used. They further determine what anthropometric measurements, lab data, and food-related measurements should be used in the nutritional monitoring and evaluation.

31. D: Patient with at least five to six feet of functioning small bowel. When food and fluid intake by mouth are not sufficient to maintain the patient in a balanced nutritional state, enteral nutrition therapy may be considered. There is considerable evidence that enteral nutrition support preserves mucosal immunity in critical illness. The underlying mechanisms maintain not only gastrointestinal mucosal immunity, but also pulmonary mucosal immunity from bacterial and viral infections. Higher rates of infection are seen with parenteral nutrition support. A patient needs only two to three feet of functioning small bowel to absorb nutrients. If there is any less bowel, parenteral nutrition support must be considered.

32. C: 30-40%. Standard enteral nutrition support formulas typically contain 30-40% of their kilocalories in the form of lipids. Lipids in the formulas are usually from corn, soy, sunflower, safflower, or canola oils. Approximately 2-4% of the daily calories should be in the form of linoleic acid to prevent essential fatty acid deficiency. High doses of linoleic acid may suppress immune function, so they are not recommended. Short- and medium-chain saturated fatty acids, monosaturated fatty acids, and omega-3 polyunsaturated acids are used in disease-specific formulas in varying amounts. Omega-3 fatty acids have been used in specialized formulas because of their modulating effect on immune function.

33. B: Alanine and glycine. Commercial parenteral nutrition solutions contain all the essential amino acids and some of the nonessential crystalline amino acids. Nonessential nitrogen is provided principally by the amino acids alanine and glycine, without aspartate, glutamine, cysteine, or taurine. Specialized products are available for pediatric use, renal disease, and liver disease, but they are used infrequently because of their expense. In most solutions, protein ranges from 3-20% of calories and provides 100 g protein per liter. At 4 kcal per gram, protein should supply about 15-20% of calories.

34. A: 0.5-1.0 lb per week. A BMI of 27-35 represents moderately overweight through class II obesity. Theoretically, since 3500 calories represents one pound of fat, if a person subtracts 500 calories from his or her daily intake for a week, there will be a weight loss of one pound per week. This would be a sensible food intake that would encourage a reasonable weight loss and an opportunity to learn better eating habits. The goal in obesity management should be refocused on weight management, rather than achieving an ideal body weight. This means setting achievable weight-loss goals and aiming toward the best achievable weight for optimal overall health

35. D: BMI of 40 or more. Body Mass Index (BMI) is a calculated number that attempts to describe the level of body fat a person has. It is found by taking the weight in kilograms and dividing it by height in meters squared. Normal BMI is 18.5-24.9; overweight, 25-29.9; class I obesity, 30-34.9; class II obesity, 35-39.9; class III obesity, 40 or more. In the morbidly obese, where diet and exercise plans have failed in the past, more drastic measures, such as bariatric surgery, may be called for. Although there may be risks with such surgery, it is the most assured way to lose a significant amount relatively quickly and may even boost the patient's motivation to follow a nutrition and exercise plan.

36. C: Weight maintenance. Childhood obesity significantly increases the risk of obesity in adulthood, along with abnormalities in blood pressure, lipid, lipoprotein, and insulin levels. Nevertheless, the weight management goal in children is weight maintenance, rather than weight loss. The primary goal for nutrition in childhood is normal growth and development; thus, all food plans should be geared toward this end. Since severe or even moderate calorie restriction may hinder growth and development, the commonly-held belief is that the obese child should grow into his or her weight. The dietitian should develop a weight maintenance plan for the next few years until current weight is appropriate for height. Only in extreme cases would weight loss be recommended.

37. A: Autoantibodies. Type 1 diabetes mellitus is an autoimmune disease in which the body's immune system develops anti-beta-cell antibodies that destroy the insulin-producing beta cells of the pancreas. Therefore, exogenous insulin is needed for life. Insulin resistance is a characteristic of type 2 diabetes mellitus, in which there is decreased tissue sensitivity to insulin, resulting in an increased insulin requirement. Hypoglycemia or low blood sugar is seen in both type 1 and type 2 diabetes. Insulin-requiring diabetes is a condition in type 2 where the pancreas can no longer produce insulin; thus, oral medications cannot control the situation, and exogenous insulin is required.

38. D: 90-95%. The incidence of type 2 diabetes is far greater than that of type 1. Risk factors for type 2 diabetes include genetic and environmental factors, including a family history of diabetes, older age, obesity, especially intraabdominal obesity, level of physical inactivity, prior history of gestational diabetes or pre-diabetes, and race or ethnicity. Because of its slow onset and because it often lacks dramatic symptoms, microvascular and macrovascular complications are frequently seen at diagnosis. The initial treatment is often diet and exercise or oral medications, but insulin may eventually be required.

39. B: Intake of unsafe foods. Excessive energy intake is associated with overweight and obesity. Obesity is one of the primary conditions associated with type 2 diabetes mellitus. Altered GI function may be present in both type 1 and type 2 diabetes. The microvascular complication of neuropathy affects the autonomic nervous system in 60-70% of people with diabetes and can affect GI tract functioning. The most common GI condition among diabetes patients is gastroparesis— delayed or irregular gastric contractions that result in sporadic gastric emptying and feelings of fullness, bloating, nausea, vomiting, diarrhea, and constipation. Other forms of neuropathy affecting the GI tract include esophagitis, loss of nutrients in the small bowel, and diarrhea or constipation in the large bowel.

40. C: SMBG. Self-monitoring blood glucose testing (SMBG) is the best way to determine occasions of hypoglycemia. It can be used by the patient at the time symptoms occur and may detect a transient occurrence of hypoglycemia where other methods of testing would not. An A1C measures the average blood glucose over the past several weeks; thus, it cannot document hypoglycemia. A glucose tolerance test is a lengthy and sometimes uncomfortable test, which may put the patient through the unnecessary unpleasant symptoms. Fasting blood glucose measures the baseline morning blood glucose after an overnight fast.

41. C: Overweight. Body mass index (BMI) is a definition for degree of adiposity and a validated measure of nutrition status. BMI is the most commonly used height-weight ratio. Its formula is BMI = Weight (kg) ÷ Height (m) ^{2}. This patient's BMI is 28.1. A BMI under 18.5 indicates underweight. A BMI from 18.5-24.9 equals a healthy weight. A BMI of 25-29.9 indicates overweight, and a BMI over 30 connotes obesity. Over 40 indicates morbid obesity. Therefore, a BMI of 28.1 indicates overweight.

42. A: Vitamin C. The objectives for nutrition therapy in chronic pancreatitis are to prevent further damage to the pancreas, decrease the attacks of acute inflammation, alleviate pain, decrease steatorrhea, and correct malnutrition. Nutritional intake should be as liberal as possible, but some limitations and supplementation may be necessary. When pancreatic function is diminished, supplemental pancreatic enzymes may be necessary to properly digest fat and protein, prevent malabsorption, and protect against steatorrhea. Loss of fat-soluble vitamins can occur with significant steatorrhea, so supplementation is advised. Also, deficiency in pancreatic protease necessary to cleave vitamin B_{12} from its carrier protein could lead to vitamin B_{12} deficiency, so supplementation of this vitamin is necessary. There is no need for vitamin C supplementation.

43. D: Malnutrition. Moderate to severe malnutrition is a common finding in patients with advanced liver disease. This is extremely significant because malnutrition plays an important part in the pathogenesis of liver disease and has a negative impact on its prognosis. Inadequate oral intake is the major contributor to malnutrition; it is caused by anorexia, dysgeusia, early satiety, nausea, vomiting, and drugs used to treat liver disease. Malabsorption and maldigestion also play a role in the malnutrition of liver disease. Positive outcomes have been shown in malnutrition with both oral and enteral nutrition support, including improvement in nutritional status and clinical complications.

44. C: White bread. The glycemic index (GI) was developed to compare the physiological effects of various carbohydrates on blood glucose. The glycemic index measures the relative area under the postprandial curve of 50 g digestible carbohydrate compared with 50 g glucose or white bread. When white bread is used, the number is multiplied by 0.7, because the GI of glucose is 100 and the GI of white bread is 70. The estimated GI of foods in meals is determined by multiplying the GI of foods by the amount of the carbohydrate in each and totaling the results. Low GI diets obtain better blood glucose levels than high GI diets, but there are some inconsistencies.

45. D: Vitamin B_{12} supplementation. Nutrition assessment in heart failure (HF) patients has shown that 54% of nonobese individuals have malnutrition. This is a primary consideration in dietary management. Small frequent meals are recommended. In terms of dietary restrictions, it is important is to control fluid retention with a limit of 2 liters of fluid and less than 2 mg sodium per day. Because of underlying atherosclerosis, a heart-healthy diet is usually given—one low in saturated fatty acids and trans fatty acids with increased fiber, fruits, and vegetables. Supplements recommended include potassium, calcium, vitamin D, thiamin, and magnesium.

46. B: TPN. MNT is especially important in acute renal failure because the patient is suffering from uremia, metabolic acidosis, fluid and electrolyte imbalance, and physiologic stress that increases protein needs. Malnourished patient with ARF have a higher mortality rate. Because oral intake is not tolerated well and enteral feeding runs into many of the same problems, TPN often is the feeding method of choice. A solution of glucose, lipids, and both essential and nonessential amino acids is initiated, with higher proportions of carbohydrate and lipids to spare protein, and fluid and electrolytes matched to output.

47. A: Prevent uremia with significant protein restriction. In the past it was thought that protein should be severely limited in end-stage renal disease (ESRD). But thinking has changed, and protein requirement varies, depending on treatment, from .06-1.0 g/ kg before dialysis to 1.2 g/kg on hemodialysis and 1.2-1.5 g/kg on peritoneal dialysis. Nutrition care plans should be designed to prevent nutritional deficiencies from malnutrition or nutrient loss in dialysate. Fluid and electrolyte balance is also a consideration in nutritional planning, along with adjustment of calcium, phosphorus, and vitamin D to prevent osteodystrophy.

48. D: Urticaria. In HIV, the combination of the disease itself and its treatment may cause a number of metabolic/medical complications. Insulin resistance and elevated blood glucose are often seen in individuals with HIV, in a great part due to medication side effects. Oral hypoglycemic agents and even insulin may be needed to control the onset of diabetes. Dyslipidemia is frequently present, including elevated triglycerides, increased LDL, and low HDL. This necessitates a diet high in fiber, fruits, and vegetables and low in saturated fat and trans fatty acids. Osteoporosis is also frequently present, due to low body mass, wasting, hormone deficiency, and previous corticosteroid use. Drug therapy may cause greater bone turnover and loss of mineral density. Supplements of calcium and vitamin D are necessary, along with a calcium-rich diet. Urticaria is an allergic skin reaction not usually associated with HIV.

49. B: Omega-3 fatty acids. Sixty percent of the brain's dry weight is fat, and twenty-five percent of this is docosahexaenoic acid (DHA), an omega-3 fatty acid. In fact, omega-3 fatty acids seem to be the substrate preferred by the brain and nervous system. They are the brain's building blocks, providing a structure for neurons and an anchoring point for neurotransmitter receptors. Eicosapentaenoic acid (EPA), another omega-3 fatty acid, can be converted to DHA. Both are found in fish and algae. Omega-3 fatty acids may also have anti-inflammatory and antioxidant effects on the brain.

50. C: Waist circumference. Waist circumference measures abdominal obesity, an important risk factor for metabolic syndrome, heart disease, and diabetes. The measurement is taken below the rib cage and above the umbilicus. A measurement of greater than 40 inches for men and 35 inches for women presents a risk factor. Regional fat deposits are genetically determined, so the tendency toward abdominal obesity is inherited. This is called android or "apple-shaped" obesity, and is most often seen in men, but can occur in women as well. This type of obesity is highly related to insulin resistance. The other type of obesity, not related to insulin resistance, is pear-shaped obesity, where fat accumulates in the hips, buttocks, and thighs.

51. A: Psychosocial behavioral analysis. The models for behavioral change describe the method of education and counseling used by the RD. The most common models include the transtheoretical model (TM) or stages of change, cognitive behavioral therapy (CBT), and motivational interviewing (MI). TM describes change as a process where individuals advance through six stages of change. These six stages of change are

1. Precontemplation
2. Contemplation
3. Preparation
4. Action
5. Maintenance
6. Relapse

The counselor determines the stage of change and uses the change process matched to that stage. CBT assumes that thinking determines behavior and relative beliefs may be identified and altered to cause a desired change in thinking and thus change behavior. Motivational interviewing (MI) can be used to help clients recognize their problems and begin to resolve them. The goal is to increase intrinsic motivation so clients can express rationale for change. Persuasion and support are the needed input from the counselor.

52. C: Education level. Understanding elements that deter or facilitate change is essential for effective nutritional counseling. People make behavioral changes only when they are ready. It is up to the RD to determine the patient's readiness or resistance to change and act accordingly. The nutritionist's style also affects the willingness to change. The RD should be positive, culturally sensitive, and empathetic, and should avoid arguments and defensiveness while supporting self-efficacy. Patients may display ambivalence. As they think about their lifestyles and certain situations in their lives, they may see behavioral change related to nutrition as too difficult to manage. On one hand, they want to make the required change, but on the other, they may not see it as important enough. Ambivalence is normal, and it is the job of the nutrition counselor to present change in such a way that the patient sees it as possible. The patient's education level should not be a factor influencing their desire to change, though they may need to be educated on the benefits of such changes.

53. A: Cognitive behavioral therapy. Cognitive behavioral therapy relates thinking and beliefs to behavior. For example, the patient states that he believes he must have a big dish of ice cream every evening; it is soothing, it makes him feel good after a tough day at work, and it helps him fall asleep. So, he eats ice cream before going to bed. Changing the belief, "I must have ice cream," will lead to a change in eating behavior. The counselor may ask the patient "Must you have ice cream, or do you like to have ice cream? Was there a time that you did not have ice cream and survived? Ice cream is high in calories, fat, and cholesterol. Do you really want to risk worsening your heart disease by eating ice cream? With your heart disease in mind, do you think maybe you could try to have a portion-controlled ice cream bar, rather than over a pint in a dish?"

54. C: Sequential. The child is a sequential learner and establishes a knowledge base by building one lesson upon another, often by memorization. The adult is a self-directed, goal-oriented learner and must be actively involved in the learning process. An adult will look at the goals and objectives of the teaching before it starts and decide if he or she wants to meet them. The adult is also relevancy oriented and must see the reason for learning the material as relevant to life. The dietitian must establish acceptable learning objectives that the patient sees as relevant to his or her life and medical situation and actively involve the learner in the teaching process.

55. D: Remind the patient that for health reasons it is necessary to make this change in his diet. The patient must recognize the goal of learning and see the benefit of reaching that goal in order to be motivated. The dietitian should establish an open, friendly atmosphere in which to present goals and then should offer support to reach them. He should ask the patient to describe barriers to learning— socioeconomic issues, activities of daily living, scheduling difficulties, etc.— and discuss how to deal with these barriers. The dietitian should also work any desired behavioral change into the existing structure of patient's life as much as possible.

56. B: Constructing a meal from his diabetic meal plan. Adult learners are task-directed and like to be involved in the learning process. The atmosphere should be positive. Dietitians should refrain from using value judgments, such as "bad." Memorization is a process in childhood learning when the student is building his or her knowledge base. The adult learner balks and loses interest when presented with this sort of learning activity. Developing a diabetic meal plan helps the patient relate new knowledge to daily life and enforces its relevance. It allows the patient to use this knowledge to accomplish a goal.

57. A: Persuasion and support. Motivational interviewing is an early stage in patient learning that sets the stage for what is to come. The goal is to establish motivation and help the patient to internalize it. Also, motivational interviewing should help the patient grasp and be able to explain the rationale for change. People make behavioral change only when they see the need and when they want to change, so the role of the dietitian is to present a good case for change and offer guidance and support for implementing it.

58. C: Suitable IT development. The Academy of Nutrition and Dietetics' research priorities include public health, implementation science, clinical nutrition research, and nutrition-related discovery. Dietetics encompasses the effective delivery of dietetic services, the implementation of the nutrition care process model, and nutrition interventions and outcome. Nutrition research consists of basic sciences as applied to nutrition and nutrient functions in health and disease. These priorities were established in 2018 by the Academy's Research Priorities and Strategies Development Task Force to focus dietetic research efforts towards the most relevant priorities.

59. B: Interventions to prevent and treat obesity and other chronic diseases. The rate of obesity in the United States has reached epidemic proportions; it is the highest of any developed nation in the world. Approximately 32% of Americans are overweight and over 42% are obese. Obesity in and of itself is unhealthy, but it also carries high risk factors for other chronic diseases, such as diabetes, hypertension, hyperlipidemia, heart disease, and more. The treatment of obesity is essential to our nation's health. Traditional low-calorie diets alone do not work to combat the problem. The very concept of "going on a diet" implies that it is a transitory thing and that one will eventually go off it. Treating obesity involves lifestyle change, a new pattern of eating, and exercise, which must become permanent. Research on lifestyle change and how to implement it into the obese person's life is a priority in nutrition research.

60. D: Intelligence. The vocabulary and speech pattern of the dietitian are important when approaching someone who is not fluent in the English language. The dietitian should look directly at the patient, speak slowly and clearly, and choose simple words that do not have multiple meanings. In our culture, we are taught to make eye-contact when speaking. This shows self-confidence and interest. Other cultures may find eye-contact to be threatening or disrespectful. It is important that the dietitian make an effort to determine how best to approach the individual patient. It is also important to be aware of another culture's eating habits. For example, it is common among some Latinos to use a large serving spoon to dish out portions. This spoon holds ¾ cup to 1 cup, and the dietitian will do better to describe serving sizes in terms of "spoons."

61. C: Set by the dietitian according to diagnosis. The dietitian should not set his own goals for a patient or present a standard diet plan. Everything should be tailored to the individual patient. Goals should be achievable. They should be set by the dietitian together with the patient after an in-depth discussion with the patient to determine what is realistic for the individual. Goals should short term so the patient can see results. For example, the dietitian should focus on a one pound per week weight loss, rather than a total of 50 pounds. Goals should be the basis for the action plan. The plan should be developed along with the patient to show how the goal of one pound per week weight loss can be achieved

62. A: The first session, in which the dietitian establishes rapport. It is the first session that sets the tone for the counseling relationship. The dietitian may be the patient's first contact with nutrition and patient education. Quiet and privacy are important. For example, when dealing with a mobile hospital patient, it would be a good idea for the dietitian to use a small meeting or examining room to avoid hospital activity and provide privacy. At the first meeting, the dietitian can make an assessment of the patient, taking note of his background, lifestyle, readiness to learn, and barriers to change and can then present some general information to get an idea of how to proceed.

63. C: Amylase. Amylase is secreted from the salivary glands into the mouth where its salivary form, ptyalin, begins the hydrolysis of starch. It is also secreted by the pancreas into the small intestine to hydrolyze starch and produce maltose and dextrins. Sucrase, nucleotidases, and enterokinase are secreted in the small intestine and have very specific roles. Sucrase breaks sucrose down to glucose and fructose. Nucleotidases hydrolyze nucleic acids to form nucleotides and phosphates. Enterokinase works on trypsinogen to activate trypsin to produce dipeptides and tripeptides.

64. C: 200-300 m². The absorptive surface of the small intestine is 200-300 m². It is the primary place in the gastrointestinal tract for absorption of water and nutrients. The large absorptive surface area is due to its great length and folds, valvulae conniventes. The surface area is covered with small finger-like projections, villi, which are then covered by microvilli, the brush border. The great surface area is due to all these tiny projections and the intestinal folds. The villi are set on a supporting structure, lamina propria, containing connective tissue with blood and lymph vessels that absorb the products of digestion.

65. B: Activity level. Fat free mass (FFM) is metabolically active tissue, as opposed to fatty tissue. The amount of FFM of an individual is a strong predictor of REE (resting energy expenditure). The more metabolically active tissue, the higher the REE. The sex of an individual affects the REE in two ways. First, men are larger than women and therefore more metabolically active. Men also have a greater proportion of muscle to fat, again rendering more FFM, thus a higher REE. In hormonal disorders such as hyperthyroidism and hypothyroidism, energy expenditure is higher and lower, respectively. The metabolic rate of women fluctuates with different phases of the menstrual cycle. Activity level has no impact on resting energy expenditure.

66. A: Sucrose. Sucrose is a disaccharide; it is a combination of glucose and fructose. Glucose is the most widely available sugar in nature. It is usually combined with another sugar or sugars to form disaccharides or polysaccharides. Dextrose is the glucose that results from the hydrolysis of cornstarch. Galactose is the result of the hydrolysis of lactose (milk sugar) during digestion.

67. D: Level on the glycemic index. Postprandial blood glucose is dose dependent, so it varies with the amount of carbohydrate consumed. The availability or digestibility of carbohydrate is also an important issue in post-meal glucose levels. Fiber can slow or hasten the digestion of carbohydrate, depending on its type. Nonsoluble fiber increases the water-holding ability of undigested material and speeds the transit time, making carbohydrates available sooner. Soluble fiber, on the other hand, can form soluble gels, increasing transit time and thereby slowing transit and decreasing nutrient absorption. After digestion, glucose enters the portal vein for transport to the liver, where depending on physiological circumstances, it is absorbed. Then glucose is available to the bloodstream for insulin-dependent absorption by tissues. The amount of available insulin and any insulin resistance will affect glucose uptake.

68. C: 50%. After carbohydrate in ingested, digested, and broken down to monosaccharides in the small intestine, it is transported via the portal vein to the liver. In the liver, glucose is available for oxidation and storage as glycogen. Galactose and fructose are also made available for the glucose metabolic pathways. About 50% of glucose is absorbed by the liver.

69. B: They influence neurotransmission. Omega-3 fatty acids are found in marine algae and consumed by fish. By eating fish, humans ingest omega-3 fatty acids. Omega-3 include docosahexaenoic acid (DHA) and eicosapentaenoic acid (EPA), which converts to DHA. These long-chain fatty acids form the brain's structure. DHA is preferred by the brain and provides structure for neurons and, among other things, is the substance that provides and maintains the density of dopamine and serotonin neurotransmitter receptors; thus, it is crucial in neurotransmission and may be essential for the effectiveness of antidepressants.

70. D: The presence of free radicals. Vitamin E is a fat-soluble vitamin, the fundamental role of which is as an antioxidant protecting the cell membrane from free radicals. Vitamin D absorption takes place in the upper small intestine by micelle-dependent diffusion. Its absorption and use are dependent on dietary fat. Also necessary for proper absorption is a fully-functioning pancreas producing pancreatic enzymes, as well as an adequately functioning liver. In the liver, vitamin E is incorporated into VHDL by use of a transport protein that is specific for vitamin E. In the bloodstream, Vitamin E is also incorporated into LDL and HDL, where it may protect these lipoproteins against the oxidative process.

71. A: Alcohol. Thiamin is essential in carbohydrate metabolism and neural function. It is activated by phosphorylation into thiamin pyrophosphate (TPP), its functional form. TTP is a critical coenzyme for several dehydrogenase enzyme complexes. It is one of these enzymes, alcohol dehydrogenase (ADH) that metabolizes alcohol in the liver to acetaldehyde. Subclinical thiamin deficiency may develop in those with excess alcohol intake who have a higher demand for thiamin and impaired absorption. Physical damage related to thiamin deficiency occurs before overt signs appear. The final stage in the progression of thiamine deficiency in heavy alcohol use is known as Wernicke-Korsakoff syndrome, which may cause a range of symptoms from mild confusion to coma.

72. C: Folate. Folate acts as an enzyme substrate in many of the body's synthesis reactions in the metabolism of amino acids. Due to the interaction of folate and vitamin B_{12}, the absence of sufficient vitamin B_{12} can cause secondary folate deficiency. In this case, folate is entrapped in a metabolically useless form, resulting in a deficiency. Folate is necessary for the synthesis of methionine from homocysteine, a process that also requires vitamin B_{12}. If methionine cannot be synthesized from homocysteine, homocysteine accumulates in the blood. High serum levels of homocysteine have been associated with atherosclerosis and heart disease. Folate is especially in important in the synthesis of fast turnover cells, such as red and white blood cells in bone marrow. Insufficient B_{12} impairs this process, causing megaloblastic anemia.

73. A: Ascorbic acid. The efficiency of iron absorption relates not only to its source food but to foods consumed at the same time. Ascorbic acid is the strongest facilitator of the absorption of iron. It helps keep iron in its ferrous or usable state. Vitamin C helps form soluble compounds with iron that render it in an available form, even in the alkaline pH of the lower intestine. In addition, ascorbic acid forms soluble compounds with phytates and tannins that bond in their normal state to prevent the absorption of iron.

74. D: Low fiber diets. Availability of calcium depends on the form of the calcium in foods and the interaction among foods consumed concurrently. Vitamin D and lactose enhance calcium absorption; phytates and oxalates that bind with vegetable sources of calcium inhibit absorption. Thus, a diet rich in dairy products would increase availability of calcium, whereas a high fiber diet rich in phytates and oxalates would decrease it. Calcium absorption seems to decrease with age. Although normal middle-aged adults adapt to a less- than-desirable calcium intake by increased absorption, this adaptability is decreased with age. Hormones such as thyroid, parathyroid, growth hormone, and estrogen can also affect calcium absorption.

75. B: 9 g/day. The high nutritional needs in infancy are based on rapid growth and development. Adequate nutrition is as crucial for brain development as it is for growth. Also, it has been reported that excess calories deposited as fat during the first 18 months may lead to the development of extra fat cells that remain for life. So, it is essential that infants receive high quality nutrition with the emphasis on protein. Nutritional requirements for this stage of life are patterned after mother's milk, as this is the most desirable form of food. Human milk supplies only six grams of protein, but it is believed that there is better absorption of amino acids from this source. Therefore, the requirement that that allows for formula feeding is higher, at 9 grams.

76. D: 1700-1900

Food	Amount	Calories	Protein	Carb	Fat
Pasta	1 c	186	6		
Dinner roll	2	172	4.8	28.6	2.1
Chicken leg	2	408	42		22.8
Alfredo sauce		172		28.6	4
Salad dressing	2 tbsp	180		4.6	13.4
Broccoli	1c	44			
Butter	3 tsp	135		8	13.4
Greens					
White wine	10 oz	200			
Coffee and ½ & ½	2 tbsp	39		1.3	3.5
Choc. ice cream	0.5 c	165		15	10
		1701	52.8	86.1	69.2

77. B: 51-85. (Please refer to the above table for calculations). Restaurant meals typically have more fat and calories than those prepared at home by a careful cook. At home, rolls and butter are not frequently served with dinner. Here, rolls and butter account for extra calories and fat. Restaurants also routinely prepare and serve vegetables with added butter. Meat and poultry are prepared for taste, not nutrition, and fancy sauces may be the rule, rather than the exception.

78. B: FIFO. FIFO stands for First In First Out. It describes a storage and stock rotation principle that ensures that goods are used in the order in which they were delivered. In effect, the first lot of a product that was delivered and came into the storeroom would be the first taken out of the storeroom and used. This keeps the latest delivery in the back of storage area or shelf and allows for the older delivery to be placed in the front and used first. As the first supply is used, the next moves up to the front, and a new delivery would be placed in the back. So, the stock is rotated according to its age.

79. A: Labor. Labor is a variable cost. Variable costs depend on the number of meals served. If the number of meals served increases, labor will be directly and immediately affected, since more meals require more employees to prepare and serve them. Initially, this would likely mean overtime pay for some of the current staff, who would have to stay extra hours or come to work on days off. Eventually, if the increase in meals served were to persist, new employees would have to be hired in permanent positions to accommodate the increased work load, and labor costs would rise.

80. D: Decreasing transit time between preparation and serving areas. An ideal storage area should be located so that labor requirements for issuing items and transit time between storage and preparation areas are minimized. The storage room should be positioned so delivery and receiving time and labor requirements for those tasks are kept to a minimum. The storage room should not be located where anyone passing by could enter and leave without being seen. There should be no extra entrances, and the entrance that is used should be attended by a clerk at all times. The location of the storage area has no bearing on transit time between preparation and service areas.

81. C: Frequently used items. Frequently used items are those that are most in demand by preparation staff and that necessitate the most trips to the storeroom. These items should be placed at the entrance of the storeroom where they can be quickly retrieved by the preparation and service staff, minimizing transit time for employees. The items delivered belong on the front of their shelves. Perishable items belong in a refrigerator or freezer. The exception is items that are frequently used.

82. D: Not leaving food out for more than 30 minutes. Food should never be left out in the open where it can be exposed to bacteria in the surrounding environment. Bacteria thrive in moisture-rich environments, so food should be kept dry. Bacteria in food grow more slowly between 40 °F and 140 °F. Heating to a temperature of 170-212 °F will kill most bacteria. Bacteria grow more rapidly at temperatures of 40-140 °F, and can subsequently cause food-borne illness. It is also essential that any employees handling food have clean hands or gloves, and that all equipment is maintained in sanitary condition.

83. B: Prevent layoffs. Labor cost control should maximize efficiency by using employees effectively to do clearly-defined jobs, following efficient procedures. In order for the employees' services to be used effectively, the job description should be presented upon hiring or update and explained, giving reasons why certain tasks must be performed. The staff member should have adequate training to perform the job, and periodic reviews should be done to ensure that each employee continues to function in a productive manner. In addition, the manager should maintain sufficient staff to get the job done without long periods of down time.

84. C: Have every employee read the policy and procedure manual thoroughly. If management establishes standards for cleanliness, dress, and behavior of employees, and standards for the quality of goods produced, employees will know what is expected of them, how they should present themselves, and how their work should be carried out. There should be no doubt left in these areas. This ensures uniformity when employees perform standard tasks. Training ensures that employees are familiar with standards and know how to perform standard procedures. Staff performance should be monitored from time to time to make certain that they continue to follow standard procedures so any problems in performance can be quickly corrected.

85. A: Age of employees. Equipment can be can be labor and cost saving. For instance, potatoes are a very common menu item used daily in fairly large amounts. Having a mechanical potato peeler can save hours of labor and save employees from an arduous task. This piece of equipment will pay for itself in labor cost saving. The same goes for a vegetable chopper, which can handle large volumes of onions, celery, and other foods used daily. These pieces of equipment provide definite cost savings to the institution. A carefully designed layout of the facilities can save numerous hours of employees' transit time by accommodating work flow and making frequently-used areas as convenient as possible. The menu directly determines labor costs by its complexity and the content of labor-intensive items.

86. D: Child care. Union contracts usually demand somewhat higher wages than are paid in nonunion companies. This is often the main reason employees unionize. In addition to higher wages, the union will usually negotiate for employer-paid life and health insurance. A standard life insurance policy is usually quite modest but will provide some money for an employee's family in the event of death. Health insurance is provided not only for the employee but also for the employee's family. This is becoming more and more costly, so some employers are insisting that employees make some contribution as well. Paid vacation is another benefit usually provided for in the typical union contract. This ensures that the employee receives a standard number of paid vacation days per year. This number of days usually increases with length of service.

87. C: Shows reporting relationships. The organizational plan or chart is a diagram showing the ranking of employees and their reporting relationships. It shows the highest position, including the name of the current title holder in a box at the top, with vertical lines connecting it to boxes below indicating the positions that directly report to the top, and so on down the chain of command. Horizontal lines connecting job title boxes show equal status, with cooperation rather than supervision being the main interaction. A thorough understanding of the hierarchy of personnel is essential when designing an organizational chart. Boxes contain only job titles and names, not job descriptions. Costs have no bearing on an organizational chart, nor do pathways of an operation.

88. D: Suggested age for the job. It is against federal law to assign an age designation to a particular job. It would be considered discrimination. Job objectives are important so the manager is aware of what each employee's duties entail. The required tasks are the steps to reach the job's objectives. They are the actual steps an employee must take to achieve the job's designated outcome. These duties, associated with meeting objectives, must be clearly defined and performance standards must be established. Standards include things such as the amount of time it should take an employee to perform a particular task, the tools to be used in accomplishing the task, and characteristics of the finished product.

89. B: Being aware of cost concerns. While being aware of cost concerns is always an issue in establishing standards and standard procedures, it is not a primary concern. Organizing the enterprise is the first task. This involves developing a clear picture of the business by answering some questions. Who are the customers? Are they hospital patients, institutional employees, customers of a restaurant, or schoolchildren? What do they expect? What is our product? How do we serve it? Identifying the customer and customer expectations can help the food service manager understand what organizational goals should be met. Thus, the food service manager can better understand what tasks must be performed so job descriptions can be articulated and employees can be scheduled to best achieve a goal.

90. C: When work standards or standard procedures have been changed. When new work standards or standard procedures are instituted, employees need training to meet these new standards or to follow new procedures effectively. When employees return from extended sick leave, unless some change has occurred in standards or procedures, training should not be necessary. Unless a new employee is hired into a new position that will affect the existing employees, no training is needed. Training should reflect needs of the organization and should not simply recur at a particular time.

91. D: Outside factors are an important consideration. Outside factors may affect an organization, but they are usually beyond its control. For instance, a food service department may be affected by the nursing or housekeeping departments, but these departments are beyond the scope of the work of food service. All systems do have a general purpose. A hospital food service may consider its purpose to serve healthy, temperature-specific, attractive, and prescription-correct meals to patients in a timely fashion. The food service is a closed environment, with goods coming in and finished products going out. All systems have subsystems that operate within them.

92. C: Orienting staff to the interaction of union policies and department practices. Policies and practices relating to union affairs are handled by union representatives. Management has nothing to do with union activities. The food service manager is responsible for the selection of new employees, usually with the help of human resources. The manager orients and trains new employees to the overall organization, the food service department, and to their specific duties. He also monitors employees to make sure that they are performing their job activities as trained and decides on the proper steps to take if they are not. Finally, although he may have a bookkeeper, the food service manager is responsible for all the financial aspects of his department, including financial reports.

93. B: Conventional, commissary, assembly/serve. In the conventional system, foods are prepared and held a short time prior to serving. This is the type of service commonly used in hospitals and needs sufficient labor and access to foods. Some prepared/processed foods may be used to limit production time and labor costs. With the assembly/serve system, all food preparation is done off-site. Frozen meals are purchased and stored, and are then assembled, heated, and served. Often, disposable dishes and tableware are used to avoid having to buy and maintain a dishwasher. The commissary-style system has a central kitchen, which may provide meals for consumers on site but also sends food to remote locations for final preparation and service. Because food is transported to multiple locations, this type of system is open to more contamination than some others.

94. A: Hazardous foods. FAT-TOM is an acronym to help remember hazardous foods. The letters stand for the following:

- F—food
- A—acid
- T—time
- T—temperature
- O—oxygen
- M—moisture

These relate to the conditions that favor rapid growth of microorganisms.

95. B: *Listeria monocytogenes*. Agents of food-borne intoxication produce toxins that can cause illness when ingested; they include *staphylococcus aureus*, *clostridium botulinum*, *clostridium perfringens*, and some molds. The most frequently seen is *staphylococcus aureus*. It is found in human skin, nose, pimples, and wounds. It can be found in meat, poultry, eggs, milk, and dairy-based products such as cream pie. There is usually no sign on the food that the toxin is present. *Staphylococcus aureus* is not killed by heat, so refrigeration is essential. Symptoms appear 0.5-6.0 hours after ingestion and include nausea and diarrhea. Listeria monocytogenes is an infectious microorganism.

96. B: *Escherichia coli*. Infectious organisms cause the majority of cases with food-borne illness. *Escherichia coli* (*E. coli*) is the most likely of these to cause illness in humans. It is found in the feces of humans and animals, so it may contaminate soil, water, and plants. *E. coli* may cause many GI disturbances from diarrhea to potentially fatal hemolytic uremic syndrome. Outbreaks have been reported due to undercooked hamburger, soft cheese, lettuce, spinach, and tomatoes. *E. coli* is destroyed by heat.

97. C: Interaction of food service employees. A food service manager should be aware of the symptoms of food-borne illness so he can identify employees or customers who may have contracted such an illness and act as a resource for hospital or school staff. It is essential that a food service manager have a thorough understanding of federal, state, and local regulations, and that they be followed. Regulations and codes set by government agencies establish minimum standards for food safety. Individual quality control standards may raise these standards. Also, the Joint Commission sets high standards for hospitals and inspects them on a regular basis. Cleaning and upkeep of equipment is essential for safe and sanitary food service.

98. B: HACCP. Hazard Analysis and Critical Control Points (HACCP) is an FDA educational program for food safety. It is the best, but not the only program of this nature. It is to be instituted after documented procedures and SOS for food handling are in place. These procedures are based on federal and state regulations. For HACCP to be implemented, the food service manager must have a thorough knowledge of hazards and critical control points (CCP). The basic components of HACCP are

- Identifying hazards and critical control points
- Establishing critical limits for CCP
- Establishing procedures for CCP
- Performing corrective action
- Keeping effective records and procedures to verify that the system is working

99. A: Federal and state regulations. In a busy food service operation, it may be difficult to make time for in-service education. Usually, there are at least two shifts of employees, and there may have to be two classes to accommodate both. When practicable, it is best to have a designated in-house educator who is skilled in principles of adult learning, rather than the food service manager, to handle this function. There is traditionally a high turnover rate among food service personnel; however, orientation should be given to each new employee to cover the basics of personal hygiene and food safety. It may be best to set a "critical mass" of new employees to determine when HACCP instruction should be given again. Required documentation has increased in all areas of healthcare and has become more and more burdensome. Unfortunately, this trend in healthcare is not going to decrease, so those involved have to adapt their work schedules to accommodate it.

100. D: 180 °F. Cleaning and sanitizing of dishes and tableware are essential to food safety and the prevention of disease. The food service manager must have a thorough understanding of these processes and should be aware of the types of soil to be removed, types of surfaces to be cleaned and sanitized, chemicals to be used, required water temperature, and kind of equipment employed. Sanitizing is a separate procedure from cleaning and usually requires higher temperatures. High heat is necessary to kill microorganisms that may cause illness. The temperatures for sanitation vary according to the equipment used. Each type has different temperature requirements to sanitize properly. Knowing your equipment is always key to food safety and sanitation.

101. B: Personnel. Personnel would fall under operational. The type of organization would be the first area to consider in menu planning. There would be vast differences among menus for a primary school, a general hospital, a long-term care facility, and a for-profit restaurant. A conscientious and objective study of the population served will have a significant impact on menu planning. Demographics to be considered would include age, sex, ethnicity, income, health status, and education. Sociocultural factors include religion, ethnicity, lifestyle, and values. Operational would include facility, equipment, budget, and personnel.

102. C: WHO. WHO stands for the World Health Organization, which sets nutritional standards for the world's population. These are generally lower than the Recommended Dietary Allowances (RDA). They are not part of the DRI, which are strictly American and carry a large safety cushion. The EAR, Estimated Average Requirement, is the figure that covers the nutritional needs of half of a healthy population. The RDA are the standards that would meet the nutritional needs of 97-98% of a healthy population and are the standards most commonly used. The AI, Adequate Intake, is the scientifically determined or observed nutritional needs when RDAs are not available. The UL, Upper Limit, is the highest safe level of a nutrient that can be consumed by healthy individuals. This is especially important in relation to supplements, which may be taken in large amounts by individuals who believe that these are beneficial.

103. A: Psychosocial. Psychosocial needs do not necessarily relate to food unless food is misused, as in an eating disorder. Demographics include gender, age, health, ethnicity, education, and income level. For example, an elderly, urban, mostly female Russian population with limited income would have different needs from a young, Anglo-Saxon, suburban population with children. The term sociocultural includes social and cultural factors, such as marital status, lifestyle, ethnicity, values, and religion. This would mean adding more ethnic foods to the menu and giving special consideration for the needs of groups such as Orthodox Jews, Seventh-Day Adventists, and Muslims, who observe dietary laws. Nutrition requirements for a geriatric population would be different from those of young adults and children.

104. C: Fats. The Dietary Guidelines for Americans do not address all nutrients; rather, they focus on some particularly problematic nutritional issues. Under the heading Food Groups to Encourage are more servings of fruits and vegetables from a wider variety of sources. Three or more servings of whole grain products are encouraged, along with at least three servings of low-fat milk or equivalent. Under the Fats category, Americans are advised to consume only 20-35% of their calories from fat, with only 10% from saturated fat, and to choose lean meats and poultry prepared by a low-fat cooking method. In Carbohydrates, whole grains are recommended, along with a minimum of sweeteners. Under Sodium and Potassium, sodium should be limited to 2300 mg and potassium-rich foods are encouraged. Lastly, the section Alcoholic Beverages advises those who drink to do so in moderation and discourages alcohol consumption in a number of groups.

105. A: Cycle. Cycle menus have two or more weeks' menus rotated or cycled throughout a specific period of time. This cuts down on repetition and keeps the food served more interesting. While the cycle menu cuts down on repetition for hospital patients, who seldom stay in the hospital much more than a week, it is repetitive enough for the food service staff to use standard procedures for food preparation. A static menu may offer several choices, but it is repeated daily. These are more common in restaurants and coffee shops. The single-occasion-use menu is primarily, as its name implies, used for a single occasion, usually a special event or a holiday. A du jour menu is literally a menu "of the day" and is rewritten daily. It is used in better restaurants.

106. C: Nutrition. Presentation is a broad concept, covering how foods appear on the plate, their sensory and aesthetic appeal, the blending of flavors, and contrasts in color, consistency, taste, texture, and shape. An example of poor presentation would be a sliced chicken, mashed potatoes, and mashed yellow squash, because it lacks variation in color and texture. Using broccoli spears as the vegetable would enhance both color and texture. Texture refers to the shape and mouth feel of food. By adding broccoli to the above meal, you are introducing a new texture. Nutrition should have been considered in earlier steps of menu planning.

107. B: Beverages. The entrée is the first item to determine for a menu. It is the main part of the meal and the most expensive. Other parts of the main course are planned around it, including either two vegetables or a starch and a vegetable. Soups and sandwiches are planned as alternates to the meal, or the soup may be an elective item with the entrée. Sandwiches may change, or the same sandwich may be offered as a substitute for the entrée. Beverages are usually standard items that do not change; coffee, tea, soda, fruit juice, and milk are common beverages.

108. D: One that includes modified diets. An extended menu includes therapeutic diets and makes provisions for several modifications of the same meal. A low sodium modification would include foods prepared without salt and would use a low sodium food in the place of a food high in sodium. A low-fat diet would be prepared by low fat cooking methods, and high fat foods like ice cream substituted with a low fat one, such as sorbet. A soft diet is modified in consistency to exclude tough meats and high-fiber foods, such as broccoli spears or mixed greens. A bland diet would omit high fiber and spicy foods.

109. B: Type of food served. The menu is a marketing tool. The design and format are what makes a menu appealing and interesting. If a menu is appealing, the customer will want to read it and will have a more positive attitude toward the food being served. The menu should be clean, with appropriate-size type and lots of white space. Too many design elements and too little white space will detract from the food being offered. Descriptive wording like fresh, green, crispy, or homemade add to the appeal of foods listed, but must be accurate. Truth-in-menu advertising has made it illegal to use misleading wording on menus, so items described as "fresh" must be fresh, and "homemade" items should be made on the premises.

110. B: Optimistic and pessimistic. Theory X and Theory Y is an earlier pessimistic/optimistic theory of leadership and management style, based on the belief that the attitude of the manager has a great impact on employees' performance. Theory X is an older "hard line" approach. It holds the belief that employees have an inherent dislike of work and will do as little as possible just to get by. Also, it holds that people do not want responsibility and prefer to be directed, and that that they need to be threatened with punishment in order to perform effectively. Theory Y is somewhat newer and is a positive approach. It holds the belief that people will naturally exert physical and mental effort to achieve good job performance, that commitment to the job depends on whether the objectives satisfy a higher order of needs, and that people will seek responsibility.

111. B: Maslow. Abraham Maslow developed a motivational theory of a hierarchy of needs, which he describes as follows: At the base are physiological needs, such as food, shelter, and clothing; safety, security, protection from harm, and freedom from fear are on the next level; social needs such as love, belonging, friendship, and acceptance are next; self-esteem needs, such as recognition, status, and achievement follow; and on the top are self-actualization needs, or reaching one's potential. Needs are only motivators if they are unmet, for it is the need that motivates. Higher needs can only be contemplated when lower ones have been met.

112. A: Having a strong sense of belonging to the organization. Managers have a strong identity as members of the organization and as protectors of the status quo, while leaders see themselves as apart from the organization and desire to implement change to the current order. Leaders question existing procedures and want to update them. They may think or say, "Just because you have been doing it that way for 25 years does not mean that it is the best way." Leaders are risk-takers if the payoff is great enough, and they are results oriented. They can relate to people in an intuitive and empathetic way, but they are also driven by the desire for personal achievement.

113. C: Having a strong survival instinct. The theory of situational management came from work done by Becker and Mouton at Ohio State, among others. This theory holds that leadership effectiveness depends on many factors, not only behavior and motivation. Effectiveness is a function of the leader relative to his subordinates, who really determine if a person has leadership skills. Situational variables are also involved. Employees look for particular traits in a leader; among other things, they want the leader to be honest, forward-looking, and competent. Other things employees want a leader to be are inspiring, intelligent, fair-minded, straightforward, supportive, dependable, and caring.

114. B: People power. French and Raven conducted a classic study identifying ways in which leaders acquire power. Power is an essential aspect of leadership. The leader has position power due to his place in an organization, and his personality may give him personal power. The study also identified other ways in which a leader can acquire power. Coercive power is the power of

88

punishment, i.e., when employees believe that the leader will punish them if they do something the leader perceives as wrong. Reward power is that in which employees believe they will be rewarded for something done exceptionally well. Expert power is that in which the employees feel that the leader has some expertise that will help them. Charismatic power is demonstrated when employees will follow a leader because they observe characteristics in the leader that deserve respect and admiration.

115. A: When quick action is required. When quick action is required, oral communication should be used, because it communicates urgency and elicits an immediate response. When employees are to be held accountable, instructions should be in writing and documented so there is a permanent record. Inexperienced employees should also receive written instructions so they can refer to them as needed. Anything quoted should also be given as a written communication so the quote will be remembered exactly as it is written. Other times that oral communications are best are when privacy is needed, or when a demonstration is required.

116. D: Organizational respect. Ethics can be defined as the rightness or wrongness of actions and the goodness or badness of these actions' objectives. Eli Wiesel once said that the ethical man is the who hesitates and asks himself, am I doing the right thing? In the history of management and leadership, the original goals were profit and productivity. In subsequent years, management theories have evolved to include ethics and social responsibility. The leader/manager must deal with several issues in this area, including employees' rights, the right to privacy, unethical behavior, and various cultural values.

117. C: The human factor. The staff creates the product and interacts with customers. It is essential that the food service manager have a positive relationship with his staff. He must be able to understand people and see their potential for growth and development. While the food service manager must follow strict operating procedures, he must also be empathetic and provide avenues for two-way communication. Communicating to employees that they are useful and highly valued leads to the efficient functioning of the department. It gives them a sense of pride, responsibility, and belonging, while encouraging a sense of self-worth.

118. B: Persuasion. The product should be unique in some way and have proprietary advantages; that is, it should be patented, copyrighted, or trademarked to prevent duplication by competitors. Place and distribution are other major factors in marketing a product or service. Manufacturing site and distribution process should be soundly investigated and established before marketing a product. Location of a private practice should be accessible, with ample parking, and should preferably be near other places customers habitually go. Establishing a price is the key to creating perceivable value in the customer's mind, and it places your services or product in relation to that of your competitor.

119. A: Target market. Missions, goals, and objectives are used to define an organization and determine what it will do. The target market is where the competition will be found. Once a business is defined, the target market must be established. The question that must be asked is, "Who is my customer?" Define the desired customer in order to identify the target market. Age, gender, education, income level, and lifestyle are all components of the target market. Also, understanding the customer's perspective will determine what benefits of a business must be stressed.

120. B: Product developer's image. The primary keys to successful product marketing include characteristics of the product, timing in the marketplace, and competitive positioning of the product. The product must have new advantages and be copyrighted, patented, or trademarked.

The target market must be ready for the product. The product must also have a competitive advantage over similar products on the market. The producer may aim at a particular target market, such as young, senior, elite, or others. Whichever target niche is chosen, the advertising must be specific for that market.

121. C: A dietitian is a spokesperson for an energy bar product. This situation violates the dietitian's code of ethics in a number of ways. The actual principles from the Code of Ethics for the Profession of Dietetics are shown below:

> *The dietetics practitioner provides professional services with objectivity and with respect for the unique needs and values of individuals.*

In this case, the dietitian did not show objectivity, nor did she show respect for the needs and values of individuals. She exhibited the bias of the food company, and by misrepresenting nutritional requirements, showed that she did not have respect for individuals.

> *The dietetics practitioner conducts herself with honesty, integrity, and fairness.*

This case showed that the dietitian let a business practice supersede honesty and integrity.

> *The dietetic practitioner promotes or endorses products in a manner that is neither false nor misleading.*

Clearly this dietitian took a position that was false and misleading.

122. D: Customer specific. Skimming is setting a very high price aimed at a small, elite, and profitable market. Examples might be an upscale gym or a personalized service in an expensive neighborhood. Trading down is the act of adding a less expensive service to an elite one to expand market share and profit. Underbidding is setting a price lower than competitors and allowing for a lower profit margin to make a business more attractive. It is often used to introduce a new business to the market.

123. B: Occupational Safety and Health Act of 1970. The Occupational Safety and Health Act of 1970 provides for improvement in workplace conditions, while the others concern the rights of workers. The Civil Rights Act of 1964 states that employers cannot deny employment on the basis of race, color, religion, sex, or national origin. The Age Discrimination in Employment Act of 1967 forbids employers from denying employment or discharging anyone because of age. The Americans with Disabilities Act of 1990 states that employers cannot deny employment to a qualified applicant with a disability. These acts ensure that groups of individuals who were once denied employment have an equal opportunity in the workplace.

124. C: Human resources. QWL refers to quality of work life. Increased employee satisfaction and productivity are the purpose of good work design. Design of work should improve work content and should aim at a safe and healthy work environment, a staff of people fit for their jobs, and efficient/effective work methods. Work design includes several subcategories, including work content, safety and health, and equipment design. Automation of many jobs has made the food service production and delivery simpler and more efficient and has resulted in better working hours. Careful delegation of some work contents can also improve work design. The addition of a healthy and safe work environment can improve both social and economic factors. Also, mechanization with appropriate equipment can provide for minimum human involvement.

125. A: Update the organizational chart. A performance improvement program looks at several factors, including environmental factors and employee tasks. The manager starts with a particular job that needs improvement. A position that requires much time and employee movement causing a bottleneck would be a good place to start. A breakdown of job details should show the following details: make-ready, actual productive work, and put-away. Each operation should be analyzed, noting procedure, equipment, motion, and time. The manager should then challenge every detail, including the what, why, and where of what is being done, asking if each is necessary.

Thank You

We at Mometrix would like to extend our heartfelt thanks to you, our friend and patron, for allowing us to play a part in your journey. It is a privilege to serve people from all walks of life who are unified in their commitment to building the best future they can for themselves.

The preparation you devote to these important testing milestones may be the most valuable educational opportunity you have for making a real difference in your life. We encourage you to put your heart into it—that feeling of succeeding, overcoming, and yes, conquering will be well worth the hours you've invested.

We want to hear your story, your struggles and your successes, and if you see any opportunities for us to improve our materials so we can help others even more effectively in the future, please share that with us as well. **The team at Mometrix would be absolutely thrilled to hear from you!** So please, send us an email (support@mometrix.com) and let's stay in touch.

If you feel as though you need additional help, please check out the other resources we offer:

> **Study Guide: http://MometrixStudyGuides.com/RD**
>
> **Flashcards: http://MometrixFlashcards.com/RD**